T0321235

STALIN AND MEDICINE
UNTOLD STORIES

STALIN AND MEDICINE

UNTOLD STORIES

Natalya Rapoport

Research Professor Emerita
Department of Biomedical Engineering
University of Utah

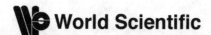
World Scientific

NEW JERSEY · LONDON · SINGAPORE · BEIJING · SHANGHAI · HONG KONG · TAIPEI · CHENNAI · TOKYO

Published by

World Scientific Publishing Co. Pte. Ltd.

5 Toh Tuck Link, Singapore 596224

USA office: 27 Warren Street, Suite 401-402, Hackensack, NJ 07601

UK office: 57 Shelton Street, Covent Garden, London WC2H 9HE

Library of Congress Control Number: 2020001574

British Library Cataloguing-in-Publication Data
A catalogue record for this book is available from the British Library.

STALIN AND MEDICINE
Untold Stories

ISBN 978-981-120-849-2 (hardcover)
ISBN 978-981-120-917-8 (paperback)
ISBN 978-981-120-850-8 (ebook for institutions)
ISBN 978-981-120-851-5 (ebook for individuals)

For any available supplementary material, please visit
https://www.worldscientific.com/worldscibooks/10.1142/11504#t=suppl

Printed in Singapore

To my parents, Sophia and Yakov Rapoport

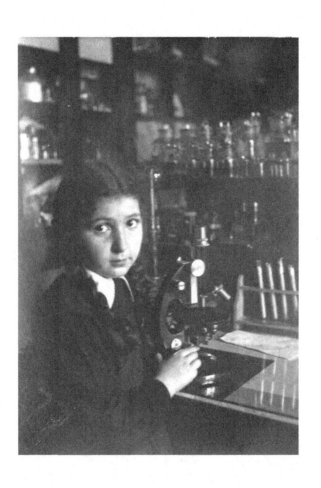

Contents

Preface

History repeats itself, first as tragedy, second as farce. These famous words have been ascribed to Karl Marx, but in fact, Marx had merely cited the philosopher Georg Wilhelm Friedrich Hegel. Many great minds have tried to discern the meaning of this maxim. The acclaimed English writer Julian Barnes expressed his doubts about Hegel's aphorism bluntly: "Does history repeat itself, the first time as tragedy, the second time as farce? No, that's too grand, too considered a process. History just burps and we taste again that raw-onion sandwich it swallowed centuries ago."

I have my own take on the subject, which stems in part from my specialty. Just as with viral diseases in individuals, a disease in society caused by a social virus, like fascism or communism, may end in tragedy — but those who survive the disease may develop the immunity needed to resist a second attack. In this way, a previous tragedy may be transmuted into farce. Unfortunately, in most cases such acquired immunity does not last long. Subsequent generations that are not exposed to the initial viral attack remain vulnerable to it, and when it occurs, tragedy strikes again. In addition, social viruses have a tendency to spread across geographic regions and infect other countries.

Could a vaccine be developed to help generations and countries decrease the risk of disease recurring, if not eradicate it completely? The great writer Mark Twain was quite pessimistic about it and said, "man's character will always make the preventing of the repetitions impossible." Indeed, history, particularly Russian history, seems to provide ample and repeated confirmations of this concept. A 19th century Russian writer once said that the country had been created to show the rest of the world what *not to do*. Russia has rewritten its history so many times and added so many lies to it that the current generation has grown up completely confused, making it easy prey for villains and dictators.

Perhaps the closest we can come to a remedy is by preserving and teaching history, to imprint it on the memory of each new generation. I have stories to tell and I consider it my duty to share them with you, my reader. After all, history is much more than just a collection of dates, events, wars, and numbers of people killed, packed into history textbooks. It is a living, pulsating flesh. If I just told you that more than twenty million people perished in some tragic historical cataclysm, you would feel little for those millions because this number is too large to be comprehensible. But if I tell you true stories of real people, you will be able to empathize — suffer, cry, and feel their horror or their joy.

Joseph Stalin was a manhunter. In his butcheries, he killed millions of people of various professions — engineers, writers, theater critics, army generals, just to name a few. His "hunting season" went on for three decades. But when he directed his boomerang against leading medical scientists and doctors, my father among them, the boomerang suddenly returned and killed the tyrant. These events went down in history as the "Doctors' Plot." The main targets of this particular hunt were doctors of Jewish origin. Vicious propaganda nailed them as "killer doctors who were deliberately murdering their patients with inappropriate treatment." There were also rumors that medicines in pharmacies were poisoned by Jewish pharmacists. A wave of panic swept the country.

People were afraid to seek medical help; outpatient clinics and pharmacies stood empty. Mothers preferred their children to die of diseases than from poisoning by "murderous" Jewish doctors and pharmacists. Unlike Stalin's other boomerang launches, the boomerang thrown at medical doctors hit bystanders.

Fortunately, several days before the planned execution of the doctors, Stalin suffered a massive stroke. Nobody was at hand to treat him because at that very time his doctors were being tortured in the basement of the Lubyanka and Lefortovo prisons. Stalin died four days later. A month after his death, the doctors were released from prison. The media reported that the case against the doctors was fabricated by the MGB, the Soviet state security apparatus. The country heaved a sigh of relief. Life gradually returned to normal, but the seeds of the "Doctors' Plot" survived through the years and from time to time they have produced ugly seedlings.

The narrative presented below is based on first-hand accounts I gained from conversations with my father and family friends. My parents belonged to the Soviet medical elite and witnessed or participated in many dramatic events that were not known to the general public. My father was one of the leading pathologists in the Soviet Union. He lived a long life and was professionally active almost to the very end. In addition, he was a dazzling storyteller. Our family enjoyed an exquisite circle of friends at the top of the Soviet intellectual society during the 20th century. Having been blessed to live for over a half century at their side, I have recorded and preserved their stories in memory, and donated documents, papers, and historical materials from my archive to the Hoover Institution in Stanford University.

"The generations of Rapoports were tied to one another in an easy, undramatic way. Their stories, even their sentences, elided xiv *Stalin and Medicine: Untold Stories*

into a single line of thought and memory. Their family narrative was nothing less than the Jewish experience in the Soviet Union in this century." — wrote David Remnick in *Lenin's Tomb*. If through these stories the reader gets a deeper understanding of the destructive effects of totalitarian regimes on society, science and medicine, I would consider my mission fulfilled.

Acknowledgments

My friends have often asked, "Why don't you write down the stories you've told us?" But my head was filled with experiments, grants, my lab, students, and mice. The development of a new technique for the targeted delivery of anti-cancer drugs has become my life's work. Seven years after my official retirement, I am still involved in it. Fortunately, there are plenty of younger, dedicated scientists who are more than capable of continuing my work, but there is no one else who can tell the stories I know. Finally I sat down to write… and immediately ran into a problem. My English proved largely sufficient for navigating daily life in the United States and for my scientific work, with its own structure and jargon, and its own set of terms of art and clichés. But this sustained, literary narrative I had embarked on clearly called for more, and I would have given up but for the help of several friends who encouraged me and agreed to read, critique, and edit my manuscript.

Dick Koehn, former Vice-President of Research at the University of Utah and the CEO of a pharmaceutical company, was the first person to read some of these stories, and I am endlessly grateful for all the red ink on the pages that came back to me.

Daniel Mattis, a renowned physicist, read the whole manuscript. I greatly appreciate his insightful critique and valuable suggestions.

My thanks also go to *Michael Clurman*, the son of my close friends Morton and Frances Clurman, the precious couple who tried to help me smuggle my father's underground manuscript from the Soviet Union to the West. Michael provided a substantive critique of the format of the manuscript. The chapter entitled "The Mystery of Stalin's Wife's Death" owes its current format — that of a courtroom drama — to him and to my friend *Alan Horowitz*, a freelance writer who suggested that I re-watch Akira Kurosawa's film *Rashomon*, which won an Academy Award in 1952.

My friend *Lynn Franklin*, a retired literary agent, read the whole manuscript and made several very helpful comments.

I also greatly appreciate the perceptive critique given by my friends *James and Julie Elegante*. James speaks many languages; he is fluent in Russian and appreciates nuances of the language, which is an invaluable asset to my cause. James is also a lawyer, and as a lawyer, he has a special eye for hidden but important formulation problems missed by other readers. Finally, James is a passionate and experienced pilot, and I am grateful to him for much more than just the editorial help. If it were not for James's expertise in piloting, perhaps you would not be reading these notes right now. Once he invited me for a flight over the Grand Canyon, and on our way back we ran into a horrifying thunderstorm. For the first time in my life I was sort of praying, but it looked like James had a sixth sense that enabled him to thread his way between the lightning strikes. Thank you, James Elegante!

Our Salt Lake City Rabbi *Fred Wenger*, upon reading an early draft, noted that it did not include any information about the author. This resulted in Chapter 1 entitled *About the Author in Her Own Words*.

Finally, this book would not exist without the help of *Marie Cochran*, who translated some chapters of the manuscript from their original Russian and polished my English in the other chapters.

Thank you, my dear friends, for all your help and for being in my life.

PART I

I *Am* Rapoport

1

About the Author in Her Own Words

When one approaches eighty, the past seems clearer and brighter than yesterday. Events that seemed trivial and meaningless bubble up to the surface and merge with other events, strung together on invisible threads like beads into a necklace, forming that which we call our destiny.

I wake up in my American home — a blessing so great that occasionally I still wake up in the morning in fear that this has all been a dream. To make sure it is for real, I go into the living room. A mountain with its brilliant cap of snow shines through the great glass trapezoid of my living room window. I have admired this view for close to thirty years and have never gotten tired of it. I have always dreamed of living in the mountains, and life has given me this unexpected gift; yet even that is a mere trifle compared with the main, the greatest gift: that I live in America. A Research Professor Emerita in the Department of Bioengineering at the University of Utah, I have spent over twenty years doing research in the field of cancer which I could not even dream of in my native Russia. How did I come to be in this Wonderland? Who am I? The depths of my memory serve up strange, unexpected episodes.

1. A Lesson in Ethics

Alyosha is my kindergarten classmate; his mother and my parents all work at the Academy of Sciences. His mother is secretary to Lina Stern, a world-renowned scientist in the field of blood-brain barriers; my mother is a senior researcher at Lina's lab. She is working on her doctor's thesis,[1] and Alyosha's mother types it up for her. This is the first draft, and my mother spends her evenings correcting the manuscript, crossing things out and writing other things in. I interpreted it as a problem with Alyosha's mother's typing: if she were a better typist, mama wouldn't have so much to correct and might have some time left for me.

"Your mom can't type," I tell Alyosha at kindergarten. "My mom keeps crossing stuff out."

Alyosha's fist delivers one of my first lessons in ethics. I tumble down the stairs, busting my knee so badly that my parents have to be called.

"He went easy on you," says my father without a trace of sympathy while my mother bandaged my knee.

Later, she explains to me my error in both its factual and its ethical aspects. Since then, I have tried, whenever possible, not to offend people.

2. My Mother, Lina Stern and the Blood-Brain Barrier

I am fortunate to have been born to a wonderful family. My parents, outstanding medical scientists, were the kindest, most intelligent, honest and courageous people I have ever encountered.

My sister and I were fond and proud of our dad but were closer with our mom. I adored her, cherished every moment she

---

[1] This was for the Doctor of Science (D.Sc.) degree, which is a one step above the Ph.D. in both the Russian and European systems.

donated to me, and always longed for more. But Mom was very, very busy with her work.

My mother was a medical scientist and a physiologist. She spent her scientific career working with Academician Lina Stern. Although I later came to appreciate and respect Lina, I was afraid of her when I was little. She was short and stout, with a sharp tongue. Born into a family of wealthy Latvian Jews, she received her medical education in Switzerland and in 1917 became the first female full professor in the department of biochemistry at the University of Geneva in Switzerland. Eight years later, her adventurous character brought her to the Soviet Union: she was captivated by the idea of helping to build the most progressive society on Earth. In the USSR, Lina became the first woman to be elected to the Soviet Academy of Sciences.

As a specialist in the blood-brain barrier (BBB), Lina was convinced that brain diseases were notoriously resistant to therapy because intravenously injected drugs could not penetrate the BBB. She suggested bypassing the BBB by injecting drugs into the spinal fluid. Around that time a ten-year old daughter of my parents' friends contracted tuberculosis meningitis, a lethal disease. Under Lina's guidance, my mother and her colleagues injected the new antibiotic, streptomycin, into the girl's spinal fluid, thus bypassing the BBB altogether. The little girl survived! It was the first such cure in the world. Unfortunately, at that time no one knew the correct dosage of streptomycin that should have been used. This drug affects the auditory nerve and as such the girl lost her hearing — but she survived!

In 1946, streptomycin was a rare drug that had just recently been developed in America. Its distribution and use were under strict government control. Of course, streptomycin was not available in the USSR, but Lina managed to get some of it through her brother who lived in America. It is not clear how he had obtained it; probably on the black market. Regardless, he sent it to her.

Lina published a paper describing the first successful cure of tuberculosis meningitis. Of course, it was not difficult to trace where this rare medicine had come from, and Lina's brother ended up in serious trouble in America and had to go back to Switzerland.

The story of the little girl's miraculous cure spread all over Moscow. Soon after, Stalin's daughter, Svetlana Alliluyeva, contacted Lina to ask for some streptomycin for her friend's daughter who had contracted pneumonia. Lina turned her down: she had very little streptomycin left and needed it to continue her research. Shortly after that in early 1949, Lina was arrested as part of the case against the Jewish Anti-Fascist Committee (JAC), one of Stalin's concocted imaginary plots. Most likely, Lina's arrest had nothing to do with Svetlana Alliluyeva's visit. Lina's Institute of Physiology, where my mother worked, was closed.

On August 12, 1952, all the members of the JAC were executed except Lina, who was spared for an unknown reason (Stalin himself had crossed her name from the execution list). There were rumors that Stalin thought she knew the secret of longevity.

Lina spent five years in prison and in exile and was released three months after Stalin's death. She spent the first several days after her return staying with us in our apartment and, sharing with my parents her recollections of those five years. The inset photograph shows my mother and father with Lina on the day of Lina's return from exile.

Soon after her release, Lina developed severe memory loss and forgot all about her arrest, imprisonment, and exile. Interestingly, she retained her sharpness of mind in scientific research.

Lina had no family and was totally dedicated to her work for which she sacrificed marriage. This sacrifice was real. As I later learned, she once had been in love with a British professor and they were engaged. My father was in scientific correspondence with this person not knowing

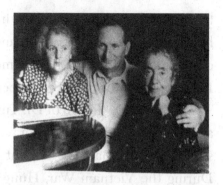

Author's parents with Lina Stern on the day of Lina's return from exile, June 3, 1953.

that he was Lina's former fiancé. One day Lina saw a letter from him on my father's desk. She recognized the handwriting and got very excited. That is when she conveyed to my father the story of her failed marriage. As it turned out, her then husband-to-be had traditional views of family life and expected her to end her scientific career once married. Lina broke off the engagement and left for the Soviet Union, but remained true to her love.

Jumping sixty years ahead, I must relate the story of a stunning coincidence that occurred in 1986 in Debrecen, Hungary. It was my very first business trip abroad from the Soviet Union. First, a bit of background. One of the facets of Soviet anti-Semitism was the all-but-official ban on Jewish scientists (and other professionals) traveling abroad on official business. When Mikhail Gorbachev came to power, this government stance, though it was not completely abolished, began to slowly be relaxed. Small changes were becoming clearly evident. After a long and vicious fight with the Communist Party organization at the research institute where I worked, I finally got permission for a three-month working trip to Hungary. More than three years previously, my scientific Hungarian colleagues had given me a standing invitation to visit and work in their labs in Budapest and Debrecen; they had steadfastly rejected other candidates that my institute had recommended to them as being "more suitable." Thanks to Gorby's Perestroika, I was finally given permission and a passport to travel.

I worked in the lab of Dr. Tibor Kelen on a three-month work assignment. Another foreigner worked in Dr. Kelen's lab, a French scientist of Vietnamese descent by the name of Hung Nguyen. During the Vietnam War, Hung and his sister escaped Vietnam in a small boat and miraculously made it to safety. They settled in Paris where both received excellent education. Hung became an assistant professor at a Paris university while his sister married and moved to the U.S.

During our term in Dr. Kelen's lab, a third foreigner, British professor Peter Plesch from the University of Keele, along with his wife Trudy, came for a short visit. A tall, elegant, silver-haired man, Professor Plesch looked distinguished. His wife Trudy matched him. We learned that Trudy received the title of Dame from Queen Elizabeth for volunteer work done on behalf of Soviet Jews. This title fitted Trudy well: she looked a real Dame.

Our Hungarian host invited us for lunch in a small private room at the University restaurant. I was seated next to Trudy Plesch, who looked at me very closely and finally asked if I was Jewish. I confirmed it, which made her really excited. I was the first Soviet Jew she had ever met. She bombarded me with questions. Her husband joined our conversation by asking me about my parents. I told him that my father was a highly recognized pathologist and my mother was a physiologist who worked with Lina Stern. Professor Plesch reacted in astonishment upon hearing Lina's name.

"Lina Stern?! You knew Lina Stern?!"

"Yes, I did. She went through my whole life, from my early childhood. Why?"

"My father was in love with Lina. Lina and my father were engaged. I could have been her son but Lina broke off the engagement and left for the Soviet Union. My father finally married my mother and they had me. But he really loved Lina. He tracked her professional publications, her social and scientific progress. Then, soon after the end of WWII,

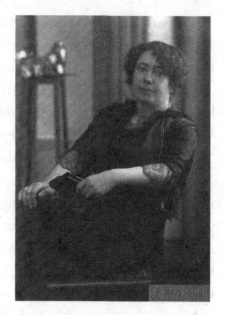

Lina Stern in her youth.

Lina disappeared from academic circles and my father could not get information about her. Even Lina's brother who lived in Switzerland had no information on her. By the way, my father was a personal doctor to Albert Einstein and wrote his memoirs about Einstein."[2]

Peter Plesch became very animated: "Please, Natasha, tell me, tell me everything you know about Lina Stern! Believe me, it is very important for me!"

And so I obliged this request from Peter Plesch and told him about the major events in Lina's life after WWII detailing her arrest and miraculous deliverance.

---

[2] Some Reminiscences of Albert Einstein. Janos Plesch and Peter H. Plesch *Notes and Records of the Royal Society of London*. Vol. 49, No. 2 (Jul., 1995), pp. 303–328 (26 pages) Published by: Royal Society

Upon later reflection, I was amazed at this coincidence. A subtle trace of Lina's only love suddenly materialized sixty years later in this provincial Hungarian town.

Our third foreigner, Dr. Hung, also had a story to tell. As he joined the conversation, Professor Plesch said, "We have a Vietnamese in our family; my nephew married a Vietnamese girl." "Yes," said Dr. Hung, "your nephew married my sister!"

This was unbelievable! His sister married Professor Plesch's nephew! The previous year, Hung and the Plesch family met at the wedding in Washington DC, but Professor Plesch did not recognize Hung until he showed his sister's wedding photographs with the Pleschs in them! Dr. Hung had known from the start of this meeting that he and the Pleschs were related but he waited for the right moment to open his cards.

Let me sum it up. Three people from three different and widely separated parts of the world meet unexpectedly in a small room in a provincial Hungarian town. And in less than two hours, they find themselves tied by invisible threads as though the world was no larger than a soccer ball...

Now back to Lina Stern. She was talented and brilliant but also extremely domineering and hard to get along with. She demanded that her colleagues match up to her own total dedication to work, but others had husbands, wives and kids. After our return from wartime evacuation and until my mother was able to put me in a kindergarten, she took me along with her to work, mortally afraid that Lina would discover me. I spent part of my early childhood in a laboratory cupboard that was specially emptied for me to hide in whenever Lina entered. (Was it then that my interest in the natural sciences was born?) Quietly sitting there in the dark, I listened to the sounds of the laboratory: the buzzing of an instrument recording the rhythms of frogs' heartbeats and muscular contractions; the clicking of thermostats; Lina's shrill voice, swearing at her colleagues.

Once, my mother had enough and said to her: "Lina Solomonovna, please don't swear at the senior scientists in front of the juniors; it undermines our authority. Take us to your office and curse there as much as you like."

"But by the time I reach my office all my anger will have evaporated," replied Lina. Her office was only two steps away, but that was what Lina was like.

My father did not share some of Lina's scientific ideas. Lina was not one to accept criticism and her relationship with my father was often rather strained, which positioned my poor mother "between two fires." She literally divided herself between work and family, which she loved to the point of complete self-denial. Unfortunately, I was a sickly child — a legacy of my cold and hungry infancy and early childhood in wartime Siberia.

"Sophia Yakovlevna, why does Natashenka get sick so often?" childless Lina used to ask accusingly. "Perhaps you don't pay enough attention to her."

Not enough attention? That was rich, coming from her; Lina and the institute already took up at least three quarters of Mama's time and they were also always trying to take the rest.

A vital detail: Lina and I were born on the same date, 26 August, exactly sixty years apart. And for a certainty, my mother would inevitably find herself having to leave my birthday parties midway for Lina's. From my celebrations, which my friends and I had planned all summer with games, songs, and performances in which I was the star, to those dull old people whose life was almost behind them.

I was about ten years old when Lina suddenly disappeared from my life; just vanished totally (as the reader recalls, Lina was arrested by the MGB). My parents answered my questions in a very evasive manner and I didn't press. Without Lina, my life became much better. Now my mother belonged to me completely; there was even a period of time when she didn't go to work. Of course, I saw that my parents were terribly discouraged by Lina's disappearance, but secretly, deep in my heart, I relished the new situation. Now, when I became ill, my mother was there at my bedside; she read to me from wonderful books and even played games with me. It was a joy to be sick!

If my ailment had gone on for too long, Dr. Miron Vovsi[3] was called. He looked at me with his kind, radiant eyes, examined me, listened to my heart, touched the swollen joints, and reproached me: "I can read it in your eyes that you had been running around again in your coat unbuttoned and with no scarf! No? Why, I know you have! Wait just a few years, you will grow up, it will all pass, and then all the puddles will be yours!"

Just a few years; easy for him to say! At that age, a few years were a major portion of my life, from which Dr. Vovsi was blithely subtracting the best part. For example, he had me excused from physical fitness lessons at school. While my whole class was excitedly chasing the ball down the hall, I had to sit on a bench by the window, utterly miserable.

Nevertheless, despite my frequent illnesses, I did remarkably well during these years. Greedily, I devoured the wisdom of the natural and exact sciences. Burning with impatience, I raced

---

[3] Dr. Miron Vovsi, my parents' friend, was a Chief Physician of the Soviet Army and an Army General. In 1952, Dr. Vovsi was arrested by the MGB and accused of being the "doctor-killer," the head of the Doctors' Plot.

through my school textbooks. Faster, faster; what's next? With delight, I attacked and solved difficult math problems. In general, I lived as though surrounded by a rose-colored screen, basking in the warm rays of my loved ones' approval. My parents wanted to keep me this way, happy and ignorant of surrounding terrors. I remained completely brainwashed by my school teachers, the radio, and newspapers, wafted along by different breezes that splashed me only occasionally with their icy spray. One event is particularly etched in my memory.

I attended Model School No. 29. During recess, the director, an old hag dressed all in black named Martyanova would plant herself in the middle of the recreation hall while the schoolgirls walked in sedate pairs along the perimeter around her. Though I was a good student and well-behaved, I was terribly afraid of Martyanova. The old woman had a collection of important titles. Delegations often visited our school to see how happily Moscow schoolgirls lived and how diligently they studied. It was from our school that Young Pioneers were chosen to lead the annual May Day parade. We were supposed to run ahead of the other marchers to Lenin's Mausoleum to present flowers to members of the government and to Comrade Stalin himself.

Excited to the depths of my patriotic soul, I even composed some verses:

> Take courage, comrades: we're the best!
> Stand up and let's away.
> For this fine group of Pioneers
> Will lead the march today!

I was going to be included in that column of Pioneers. Not even in my wildest dreams could I imagine such joy, to stand on the Mausoleum's reviewing stand, right next to Comrade

Stalin. My triumph knew no bounds! I boasted incessantly to my neighborhood friends, to my relatives, and to those friends of my parents who hadn't yet been arrested. In my wild dreams I saw myself on the lap of Comrade Stalin, replacing the lucky girl on his lap looking at us from the iconic photograph that decorated the walls of every kindergarten and school in the country.

But then the inconceivable happened. On the very eve of the celebration, just one step away from unutterable happiness and glory, my father with his sharp pathologist's eye discovered inflamed tonsils in my throat (but didn't I *always* have inflamed tonsils?). He pronounced me sick, sent me to bed, and wouldn't let me out. This was preposterous! Hadn't Papa forced me to go to school that time when I faked a sore throat because I had wanted to stay home to read an interesting book? I nearly drowned my parents with my tears, but Papa, normally so amenable, was adamant this time. And so my great dreams were shattered, leaving an ugly scar of resentment toward my parents in my childish soul. Much later I learned that my parents had known about the tragic fate of the parents of the girl on Stalin's lap: her father was arrested and executed; her young mother was most probably murdered; she was found dead during her night shift in the hospital where she worked.

However, I remained totally oblivious to the incomprehensible nature of the times. Outside my protective screen, unimaginable horrors were occurring. One after another, my parents' friends disappeared. Even in the seclusion of our own apartment, my parents spoke their names only in whispers. I remained ignorant about these horrors until one night I answered the doorbell of our apartment. But before proceeding further, I need to give you some historical perspective on the events that would become known to history as the Doctors' Plot.

3. The "Doctors' Plot" of 1953

In the last year of his life, Stalin arrested Kremlin doctors and other prominent physicians. The doctors were accused of murdering their patients — high-ranking party and government leaders — with inappropriate medical treatment at the behest of foreign intelligence agencies. Most of those arrested were Jewish, and the arrests were accompanied by a hysterical anti-Semitic campaign in the press.

Stalin's relationship with medicine was complicated. On the one hand, he used medicine as a weapon against his potential victims — he turned the Kremlin hospital into a virtual death camp, where his medically trained minions killed their patients (see the chapter "The Death Camp at the Kremlin Hospital"). On the other hand, knowing how easily medicine could be misused made him fear and mistrust his own doctors. Stalin's attending physicians always had to be on their toes.

Nevertheless, in 1952, a year before Stalin's death, his personal physician, Dr. Vinogradov, slipped up and imprudently wrote on Stalin's medical chart that Stalin had suffered multiple micro-strokes and must retire from all political activity. Lavrenty Beria, chief of the secret service, showed Stalin this diagnosis. Stalin, enraged, arrested Dr. Vinogradov and several other leading Kremlin doctors.

Mikhail Ryumin, Deputy Chief of the MGB and chief investigator for Specially Important Cases, saw it as his chance in the power struggle against his boss, Viktor Abakumov, the Minister of State Security, whose job Ryumin coveted. Exploiting Stalin's paranoia toward doctors as well as his distrust of Soviet Jews after the creation of the State of Israel, Ryumin wrote a letter to Stalin announcing the existence of a conspiracy of Jewish doctors to murder the leading Soviet officials and Comrade Stalin himself, which had been purportedly disclosed to him by the previously arrested Dr. Yakov Etinger during an interrogation. Although Ryumin's information could not be verified, Dr. Etinger having conveniently died in his cell, his plan worked: Stalin immediately arrested Abakumov and promoted Ryumin to the position of Deputy Minister of State Security. This marked the beginning of a wave of arrests of leading Jewish doctors and a massive anti-Semitic campaign. What began as Stalin's revenge against his personal physician then grew and assumed global proportions, threatening to bring about a "final solution of the Jewish question" in the USSR. That is, the death of millions and a total extermination of all Jews in the Soviet Union and its satellite countries.

On January, 13, 1953, the world was stunned by a news release published in all major Soviet newspapers:

> **Vicious Spies and Killers Masquerading as Professors and Physicians**
>
> *Today the TASS news agency reported the arrest of a group of saboteur-doctors. This terrorist group, uncovered some time ago by organs of state security, had set itself the goal of shortening the lives of leaders of the Soviet Union by means of medical sabotage.*
>
> *An investigation has determined that the members of this terrorist group, exploiting their position as doctors and abusing their patients' trust, have deliberately and viciously undermined their patients' health by making incorrect diagnoses, and then killed them with inappropriate treatments. Hiding behind the high and noble calling of physicians, men of science, these fiends and murderers have trampled upon the holy banner of science. Taking the path of monstrous crimes, they have defiled the honor of scientists [...].*
>
> *Most of the members of this terrorist group [...] were bought by American intelligence. They were recruited by an arm of the American intelligence establishment, the international Jewish bourgeois-nationalist*

organization known as "Joint."[4] *The filthy face of this Zionist espionage organization, hiding its vicious actions under the mask of charity, has been utterly exposed […].*

As most of the arrested doctors were Jewish, the terrible anti-Semitic campaign unleashed five years earlier had now reached its climax. The man in the street confidently expected to see a spectacular execution of arrested doctors in the Red Square, followed by an organized pogrom and a deportation of all Jews to Siberian labor camps. Nikita Khrushchev and others in power at that time would later describe in their memoirs some details of Stalin's chilling plans regarding Jews.

My father, a world-renowned pathologist, was one of those arrested by Stalin. His execution appeared imminent. But miraculously, several days before the doctors' scheduled execution, Stalin suffered a massive stroke and died four days later. Ironically, the arrest of Kremlin doctors may have hastened Stalin's death: one of the arrested doctors was his private physician, Professor Vinogradov, who was unavailable because he was being tortured in the basement of Lubyanka prison when Stalin's fatal stroke struck.

Stalin's death on March 5, 1953 saved the lives of the doctors, their families and most of the Soviet Union's Jewish population. A month after Stalin's death, all the doctors, including my father, were exonerated and released from Lubyanka prison. Soviet newspapers reported that the "crimes" of Jewish doctors had been fabricated by the MGB.

---

[4] This is a reference to the American Jewish Joint Distribution Committee (JDC), a New York-based Jewish charitable organization that provides financial and other types of assistance to Jews all over the world. In the 1920s and 30s, the JDC provided help to Russian and Soviet Jews. The bizarre paranoia that equated charity with espionage is typical of the Soviet public discourse of the time.

A vicious struggle for power followed Stalin's death. One of the most sinister persons in the Soviet establishment, the chief of secret police Lavrenty Beria, tried to garner political capital by ascribing to himself the cessation of the Doctors' Plot. However, about two months after the doctors' release and after Nikita Khrushchev had gained ascendancy, Beria was arrested and shot, and a short period of relative liberalism known as Khrushchev's "thaw" began.

The reader may wonder how my father, a pathologist, came to be numbered among the allegedly murderous doctors: after all, a pathologist deals with people who are already dead and would not normally be expected to be able to kill anyone, at least not as part of his work. However, the prosecution figured that he might have signed false death certificates. In this scenario, for instance, his colleagues would have killed their patients and he would have then signed papers reporting that they had died from natural causes.

If that sounds far-fetched, let me tell you a story that shows what brilliant fabulists Stalin had working for him. One of our neighbors who lived a few floors down from us in the same apartment building was Mrs. G., an older lady and also a pathologist and a professor. She was the head of pathology at a Moscow hospital and she also had a summer cottage (a *dacha*) situated diagonally behind our own. From the dacha, she could see the people who came to see us and hear what they talked about. She never asked my father for professional advice until one day, a week or two before his arrest, when she came to our home and said she needed a consultation. She told us the following story: her hospital's gynecology department had just lost a patient, a young woman who had fully recovered and was going to be discharged the next day when she abruptly became terribly ill and died the same night despite the doctors' best efforts. "What did the autopsy show?"

asked my father. Professor G. described the findings. "Why, that sounds like classic arsenic poisoning!" said my father. "You must refer the case to the medical examiner. Do you know anything about her family?" "Unfortunately, I do. Her husband is a colonel in the MGB. While his wife was hospitalized, he started an affair with a nurse working in that department." "You must refer this to the medical examiner," repeated my father.

A few days later, my father ran into Professor G. in the courtyard of our apartment building. "What did the medical examiner find?" he asked. "Nothing," she replied, "I decided not to refer it to them." My father was very surprised and wondered what Professor G. could have reported in the death certificate. He did not have to wonder for long because he was arrested soon afterwards and realized during his interrogations that Professor G. was an MGB informant. When he was released, he stopped speaking with her.

Time passed and Professor G. died and was replaced with a friend of ours, Dr. S., as head of pathology. My father asked him to check the archives for the case of that deceased young patient and to see what the death certificate said. A few days later, Dr. S. came to see us, looking baffled. "Yakov L'vovich," said Dr. S., "there's no such case! I went through all the archives and nothing like this was on file. I went over to the gynecology department — they have all the same doctors and nurses still working there — and none of them can remember a young woman suddenly dying from unexplained causes. And this would have been something so extraordinary that people surely would have remembered. They all say this never happened!"

My father was puzzled and kept returning to this story in his mind for many days until one day he finally woke me up in the middle of the night: "I got it! If our case had gone to trial, G. would have testified that I was skilled enough to tell death by poison from natural death, sight unseen! Which would then prove their allegation that when I signed those false death certificates — exonerating my colleagues — I acted with criminal intent rather than from inexperience." I suspect my father had guessed correctly. But what a stage play, what an elaborate piece of fiction this was! Truly, MGB hacks had good imaginations…

I was fourteen when my father was arrested. The events of the Doctors' Plot have etched themselves in the depths of my soul for many years and I have never ceased to feel their scorching pain. They have haunted me for decades. Finally, I found a solution: to write down my account of these events as seen through the eyes of the naive and brainwashed Soviet schoolgirl I was at that time. Somehow, writing it down has helped to relieve my anguish. This is exactly as I remember these events, a small segment of my generation's history; nothing has been embellished.

4. The Catapult

4.1 *January 13, 1953*

I remember listening to the radio — for the fifth time that day. It was a habit of mine to follow the radio broadcasts with unthinking confidence and trust in the official news bulletins. Suddenly, the words that had been washing soothingly over my mind stuck; my brain refused to comprehend and accept what I was hearing. It couldn't be, it simply could not be true! The radio mentioned Dr. Vovsi, Miron Vovsi, whose gentle hands and radiant eyes had always been there throughout my childhood and my illnesses. It mentioned other doctors whom I knew. I had been an equal opportunity patient, contracting childhood illnesses within each of their fields of expertise. Now the radio was saying that all of them… all of these kind, competent people who until just recently had been

joking, laughing, hugging me at our warm and hospitable home...
that they were all murderers, monster-freaks of the human race,
evildoers dressed in white gowns, united by a single goal: to murder the leaders of the Communist Party and the government.

"It cannot be!" I burst out, looking in shock at my parents,
equally shaken. "Tell them it's a lie! Why are you standing there?!
Run and tell them that it's a lie!"

"Yes, this is a mistake," my grim-faced Mama said in an unfamiliar, choked voice, carefully choosing her words. "It is a horrible
mistake, and it will of course be cleared up soon. But you can't tell
anyone that you don't believe this, you understand me? Not a soul!
If you do, you will bring a lot of harm to your father and me, and
you" — here followed a chilling threat — "you will be expelled
from the Komsomol! Don't talk to anyone about this!"

It was easy for them to say "don't talk about it" when everywhere — at school, around the neighborhood, on the buses and
trolley cars, in the shops — there was just one topic of conversation: the bloody crimes of the newly exposed traitors. I tried to be
patient and silent, but inside I was slowly going out of my mind, no
longer certain of what was the truth and what was a lie, which end
was up and which was down. The very ground under my feet felt
shaky and I was at a loss.

Public hysteria was simmering just beneath the surface everywhere. This was a new, Soviet form of the age-old blood libel.
Because the named doctors were mostly Jewish, the man on the
street slipped easily into the old habit of cursing all Jews, not just
the specific individuals listed in the news bulletin.

How the public thirsted for revenge! As the media whipped
up these emotions, people began to refuse being treated by Jewish
doctors. There was a distinct scent of pogrom in the air. Rumors
spread that all Soviet Jews would be relocated to Siberia, to special

camps that were being built even now; all for their own protection, of course, in order to shield them from the wrath of the public. Their mass relocation was imminent.

There was widespread speculation as to which method of execution would be used on the criminals. Informed circles in my class contended that they would be hanged in the Red Square. Many wondered about whether the execution would be open to public or only to those with special passes. Some argued the latter as otherwise the mob might stampede and damage Lenin's tomb. Some were disappointed that they might not get the passes while others tried to console them by saying that the execution would surely be filmed. In the midst of this outpouring of bloodlust, I dreamed of Dr. Vovsi on the gallows and woke up screaming.

And yet, through all of this, not even for a second — not for a flashing instant — did I dream that *this* could happen to *my* father.

But it did, a mere two weeks later.

4.2 *A History Lesson*

"Rapoport, to the blackboard!"

We couldn't stand our stupid, short-legged, malicious history teacher. Grating and grinding, she dragged the creaking ship that was our class along the dried-up riverbed of her barren historical materialism. The entirety of human history, as presented by her, was reduced to a sequence of changes from one social or economic structure to another, brought on by the contradictions between productive forces and productive relations. With a ruthlessness of a vivisectionist she dissected the living, pulsating flesh of history, forcing us to examine the cadaver. But today I was very happy that she had called on me. I liked the subject: the U.S. Constitution. I had even done a bit of extra reading in preparation for today's lesson and had visited my dear Auntie Julia for additional information.

Julia and Shabsai Moshkovsky were our close family friends. We lived in the same apartment building, which was built by the medical cooperative "Medic." We had moved there in 1951 from our communal apartment. All the tenants were medical doctors who lived there with their families. Shabsai, for instance, was a corresponding member of the Academy of Medical Sciences. His wife, whom I called Auntie Julia, had graduated from Freiburg University and she was a historian and a specialist in medieval Germany. She could speak about historical figures as if she was personally acquainted with them and about historical events as if they had happened before her very eyes. I loved her stories. We were very close, and I shared confidences with her that not even my parents knew. This time Auntie Julia had told me the fascinating story of a young America. And now, in class, I repeated her tale with great pleasure. My classmates were all ears.

The history teacher gave me a C, causing an uproar. For me, a straight-A student, even a B was an anomaly. I was stunned, and my classmates were indignant. "What? Didn't she answer correctly? What did she say that was wrong?"

"No, she answered correctly," the history teacher replied defensively, "but did you hear the tone she used? Her admiring intonation, her groveling before the bourgeois West?" Suddenly she erupted in a mocking screech: "Oh, what a wonderful country America is! I think I have an aunt in America! I think I'll go live in America tomorrow!"

Stunned by the unexpected, crude insult and deeply offended by the injustice — by the teacher's wanton disregard of my hard work and earnest effort — I quickly gathered my things and stormed out of the room, slamming the door behind me. I was determined to never go to school again.

My parents were very upset. On hindsight, it is hard to believe that they could be upset over such nonsense at a time like this, when danger was looming and both of them might be arrested at any moment (as it turned out, my father was indeed arrested a few days later). They went to see my school principal, Vera Kirichenko. The principal was a mathematician and as dry and strict as her discipline. Many years would pass before I realized what a feat this woman accomplished — unbelievably, she forced the history teacher to give a public apology!

During our next history lesson, the principal accompanied the history teacher into the classroom and sat down in the last row. Looking slightly sidewise towards a portrait of Stalin on the wall, her eyes empty of expression, the teacher limply muttered, "I have reconsidered Rapoport's report given during the previous class. Perhaps there was no groveling to America in her answer. But she failed to emphasize that since the time the U.S. Constitution was ratified, many things have changed in America and that today there are no traces of the freedoms proclaimed in the Constitution. Nevertheless, I have decided to change Rapoport's grade to a B. Give me your grade book."

Taken aback by this unexpected turn of events, I handed her my grade book. This class occurred two days after my father's arrest, but the history teacher did not know she was not apologizing to Natasha Rapoport, Komsomol member and exemplary student, but to Natasha Rapoport, the daughter of a "murderer" and a "member of an anti-Soviet organization." Such are the paradoxes of history.

4.3 *A Late-Night Visit*

At the age of fourteen, I was a remarkably oblivious child. Even though many of our family friends were among those named in the official broadcast announcing the discovery of a "criminal group of killer doctors" and "murderers in white gowns," I did not anticipate any personal misfortune. But on the night of February 2 (between the two history lessons described above), my father was arrested and disaster descended on me like a tornado.

Some people are fortunate enough to grow up smoothly from childhood to adulthood, delighting in each changing stage along the way. But I was catapulted out of my childhood. The catapult was triggered by our concierge, Lucia, shattering the late-night silence of our apartment with the doorbell. As often happened in those days, my parents were out. The sudden ring at such an hour startled me.

"Who is there?"

"Natasha, open up! There's something wrong with your heating system," Lucia's voice came through the door.

I was surprised; there was nothing wrong with our heating system.

"Natasha, open the door immediately! Your radiator is leaking, the neighbors below are complaining," Lucia insisted.

I opened the door. Standing there was a gang of thugs (at least that's what I thought at that moment), so many that the landing outside could barely hold them all. One or two were in military uniforms while the others wore civilian clothes; all looked remarkably alike.

Our apartment was overrun in an instant. Pushing me aside and against the wall, they poured in like a violent stream. At the end of our hallway, this stream divided into separate streamlets that flowed into my father's study, the dining room, the kitchen, the bathroom, and even the toilet. One of the "officers" (I was convinced they were burglars in disguise) sat in the dining room, presiding over the proceedings as though he owned the place. All the others reported to him: "Bookcases — six; wardrobes — three; cupboards — two; writing desks... beds..."

I became less anxious: "They've come to steal the furniture; they aren't going to kill me after all," I reassured myself. I did not care about the furniture; to be honest, I have always resented the way my father complained about glue on the piano keys, paint on the sofa, or scratches on the table. "Maybe everything will be all right," I thought, hiding behind the sofa in my room. The only thing I prayed they wouldn't take was the piano. It was an heirloom, recovered from our bombed-out house on Starokonyushenny Lane during the war. I was only three at the time. My parents had returned from our dacha to find our house in ruins, with the piano suspended from a girder like a ghost. It could never be tuned again, but everyone liked and admired it. I felt sorry for the piano.

Strangely, the thieves seemed in no hurry at all. They examined the apartment meticulously — each corner, every inch — and I started to worry again. Any minute now my parents could return and I was terrified to think what would happen then. My father was a proud, hot-tempered man who wouldn't mind the odds against him. He would protest violently and then the bastards would kill all of us. My teeth chattered loudly and uncontrollably.

Suddenly the telephone rang, causing my heart to nearly stop, and one of the thieves grabbed me and sternly said, "Hurry up, answer the phone, but say nothing about us being here, got it?!" My legs would not obey me. The man dragged me across the floor, almost carrying me the last few feet. He lifted the receiver, thrust it against my ear and hissed, "Answer it!"

Only my parents could be calling at one in the morning. My throat contracted in a spasm and I couldn't say a word. "Natalochka, you're not asleep yet? Do we have guests? Don't worry, we'll be home soon."

It was absolutely terrifying and altogether too much for me. I fainted.

4.4 *The Search*

I had fainted so deeply that I did not hear my parents return or my father being taken away. I regained consciousness much later in the middle of the night, still in complete ignorance. Mama was kneeling next to me. Something cold and wet was on my forehead. A strange male voice asked:

"Is this your daughter?"

"Yes."

"Yours and the arrestee's?"

The arrestee? A powerful wave seized me, whirled me around, and thrashed me, breaking my bones and bearing me away from my rosy world, my happy childhood, forever. I regained consciousness the second time as the daughter of a doctor-murderer.

In our apartment, the search was in full swing. To these professionals, the job was routine, boring, almost automatic. Search every book, page by page. Every pillow, every drawer. What's this? Oh, they've found a letter from my friend Jan; we became friends in Estonia last summer. They look it over, ask if I have any more letters, and take them all away. How was I to know that Jan's father was an Estonian priest and an important leader in the Estonian church who was now in prison, and that my friendship with Jan would become one of the links in the long chain of criminal charges against my father?

What a boring job, indeed... Oh look, they've found several books by Freud, a bourgeois, Western writer. They leaf through them, muttering; they add them to the growing pile of evidence. Now they've picked up a Finnish knife, a war trophy my father used for boating. Suddenly, a sensation! Rifling through the harmless contents of our medicine cabinet, they've found a small bottle marked with a skull and crossbones and a label that said "Poison." Here it is, at last, exactly what they are after — the necessary, irrefutable evidence! Everyone looks at the man who found it with respect and envy.

"And how many people can one of these bottles put to sleep?" asks the lieutenant, the only person present at the search who is wearing a military uniform.

"You can't kill *anyone* with this," my mother tries to explain. "This is atropine, a medication for heart disease. My husband had a heart attack, and we keep heart medicines at home to be safe."

"Sure, sure, I can see what you keep it for," says the lieutenant venomously. "I can see perfectly well what kind of heart medicine you're keeping here. Just how many hearts have you stopped with this medicine?" He is happy.

My mother's explanations fall on deaf ears. They make a telephone call to inform someone of what they have found. (It is late at night but *those people over there* never sleep). They wrap the little bottle carefully in cotton wool, seal it into a small box and insert that into yet another box, which they also seal. They draw up a document stating that poison was found in the arrestee's apartment and demand that my mother sign it. She categorically refuses. They insist and threaten her. If she doesn't sign, she will have to go with them. For a long time? Forever? I am in despair. But Mama doesn't sign.

Our visitors' elation from finding the little bottle of atropine soon passes. There has been an accident: one of them has cut his finger on a razor blade, drawing blood. What rotten luck, cutting his finger in the home of a Jew, a killer doctor — the poor fellow's days are undoubtedly numbered. The man sits in the chair, paler than the white-painted walls, holding his scratched hand extended in front of him. His comrades hover around him, talking in worried tones. What is to be done? Can his life be saved?

Mama offers the distraught man some iodine to stop the bleeding and disinfect the cut. This common-sense solution produces its own paroxysm of tension among the thugs. Should they accept it or not? She says it's iodine, this Jewish woman, the doctor's wife, but who knows what's really in it? A volunteer, with courage borne out of despair, puts a drop of iodine on his fingernail. One after another, each man sniffs it. They decide not to take the risk. They phone somewhere for a car and the sufferer is taken away — most likely to a special clinic where his scratch will be treated by a trusted, dependable *Russian* doctor.

Once the search was over, they sealed the apartment, except my small room, the hallway, kitchen, bathroom, and toilet. They took Mama away, just as they had threatened. Neither she nor I knew if we would see one another again.

But Mama did return, twenty-four hours later! It turned out that she had been taken to our dacha, which they also searched from top to bottom, down to the last speck of dust. Mama later told me that upon her return she had found me crouched in the same chair in the hallway, just as she had left me. It looked to her as though I hadn't budged at all in all that time. I myself have no memory of those twenty-four hours, except for the heartbreaking howling of our poodle, Topsy. We might have howled together, a duet of fear and grief.

When Mama came back, I felt that my life had returned with her.

4.5 *The Daughter of a Killer Doctor*

I was morbidly attached to my mother. In my childhood, whenever she went away somewhere with my father, I would simply fall ill, stop eating, vomit, and feel as though I had died, until she returned. I would count the days, the hours, the minutes. I was prepared to do anything for my mother. Mama always delighted in my achievements; after she passed away, they lost all meaning for me for a long time. But during those days after my father's arrest, it was very important to my mother that my life remained undisrupted and that I continued going to school. So I did. But from that moment on, two separate fears that merged into one endless horror took over my life: the daytime fear that my classmates would learn of my disgrace and the nighttime fear that my mother would be taken away.

The nighttime fear would come at eleven and last until five in the morning. For some reason, I was convinced that she couldn't be arrested at an earlier or later time. My fear was so strong that during those hours I trembled all over as if in a fit. I even slept in a cot out in the hallway rather than in my own room, listening tensely all night for sounds; rustling on the staircase or the closing of the elevator door made me gasp in terror.

The daytime fear held me in its grip during school hours, turning me into a tightly coiled spring. Only three girls in my class who also lived in my apartment building knew my secret. Their parents sternly forbade them to breathe a word to anyone, even to their closest friends, probably thinking that they might share the same fate at any moment. And the girls were silent, although it's easy to imagine how difficult it must have been to keep such a sensational secret. The secret, desperate to come out, burned the ends of their tongues.

I mustered all my strength to appear my usual cheerful self. But then one of the three girls broke down. She took me aside during recess and said, "You don't think we're keeping your secret just so you can strut around pretending like you're one of us, do you?" Cr-r-rack! The months of pent-up tension exploded in a resounding slap that I planted on the face of my offender. In a flash, the entire class surrounded us: "What's happened?"

The girl, this youthful enforcer of social purity, stared at me with a mixture of astonishment and hate while I, barely holding myself upright on trembling legs and on the verge of fainting, could just see the awful truth swelling up in her mouth, seeping through her teeth, and about to burst from her lips right there and then… But right at that instant the bell rang, releasing me from my paralysis. I flew to class, feverishly gathered my things, and left school — perhaps forever.

4.6 *The People Who Helped*

What did we live on after my father's arrest? My mother was fired the next morning. All the money found in our home during the search was taken, along with our bonds and savings passbook. There was, I believe, a method to this madness. In our stairwell, at the courtyard, or on the street outside our house, there were always MGB agents loitering, waiting to follow Mama and me wherever we went. They wanted to see who would come to our aid so they could haul in more people, all our friends and associates, like links in a long chain that they could then use to build their case against my father. People understood this and were afraid. Neighbors averted their eyes when they met me or Mama in the street; they tried to slip by without acknowledging us.

But not everyone did that. I will never forget our neighbors, Vladimir Nikolayevich and Nina Petrovna Beklemyshev, old-school Russian intellectuals — members of the disappearing class known as the *intelligentsia*, characterized by excellent education, sterling probity and courtly manners. Vladimir was a tall, handsome man with a pointed beard, an academician who looked as if he had stepped out of a portrait of one of the great nineteenth-century scientists, aristocrats of the spirit. Whenever he met Mama in the street, he did not simply greet her — he deeply bowed to her, displaying to others a conspicuous example of courage and nobility.

His wife Nina bravely came to our apartment right after my mother's return from the search of our dacha to offer us money. My mother did not accept it because there was no way she could ever pay it back, but Nina wouldn't leave until she received Mama's solemn promise to turn to her for help at any time, day or night.

Once, I met my Auntie Julia in the street and she took me to her apartment. She fed me, questioned me about everything, gave me extra food for Mama, and quickly sent me on my way: God forbid that Shabsai should return from work and catch us — he would die of fright. Shabsai was a kind, interesting, and totally decent person who adored children and was adored by them in turn. I myself loved him dearly, although with a tinge of indulgence, finding him peculiar in many ways: he drank plain hot water instead of tea, washed his hands obsessively, ate only the freshest food, never allowed alcohol to touch his lips, and in general was extraordinarily cautious.

In contrast, Auntie Julia enjoyed a glass of wine or two at celebrations. When their son was in first grade, he filled out a school survey about the drinking habits of his parents as follows: "Father: teetotaler. Mother: drinks." A concerned teacher then came to their house and was most surprised to be greeted by a charming, refined, and clearly sober woman with a slender, intelligent face, and to see original paintings by famous artists on the walls, with dedications showing that this particular student's parents were people of high culture rather than the troubled family she had been led to expect. For a long time afterwards, Auntie Julia continued to be the target of much friendly teasing: "Julenka, don't drink so much; surely you remember what happened last time!" Now, in comparison with Shabsai's caution, Auntie Julia's act of taking me into her home smacked of heroism, and I admired her for it.

Natashka Tomilina, a girl from our apartment building who was also in my grade at school would drop by almost every day, even though she had visited only rarely before. She would take out a sandwich and an apple from her school bag: "Here, eat this for me, will you? If my mother finds out I didn't eat the lunch she packed me, she'll kill me." Not once did she glance at the sealed doors or ask why I sat on a cot in the hallway, as though a person living in a hallway on a cot was the most normal thing in the world. Natashka would take out her textbooks: "Hey, can you help me out with these physics problems? Here's the stupid stuff we studied today, take a look!" To this day, Natashka claims that she did this without an ulterior motive. What kind of fool would rack their brain to solve those silly physics or math problems when there was a simpler, more elegant and very reliable way: having me do it? She is most likely lying. She herself was an excellent student and could easily solve those "silly problems." But in any case, thanks to Natashka, I stayed abreast of school news, gossips, and the curriculum. When I returned to school, I wasn't behind at all.

The great Russian literary classics also helped us get through this difficult time. There was a bookcase in the hallway filled with the collected works of Leo Tolstoy, Alexander Pushkin, Ivan

Turgenev, Nikolay Gogol. Mama started taking them to used bookstores, returning with bread, milk, and kasha. And so we survived. But the classics were carried out of our house in suspicious-looking, bulky sacks, and someone informed on us — they thought Mama had broken into the sealed rooms in our apartment and was selling things from there. This brought on another search. This time I almost died from fright — I thought they had come for Mama. They found the seals on the doors to be intact, broke them, and immediately saw that the accusation was false, but had to verify the contents of the rooms once again, checking them off their list — while I screamed. But they didn't take Mama. They sealed everything up again and left.

And there was one family that helped us unfailingly throughout.

4.7 *The Gubers*

My mother had shared the same desk with Raya Guber in high school and their friendship lasted their entire lives; they were closer than sisters. When I was born, my mother fell ill with typhus. Auntie Raya breast-fed me along with her own daughter Marishka, who had been born two months earlier. Her husband, Andrey Alexandrovich Guber, never missed an opportunity to remind me of that fact, implying (only half in jest) that a person who had had the privilege of being nursed by those breasts ought to work harder on their character.

The Gubers (who also had a son, Shurik, a year older than me) were my second family. Andrey was an inventor and the soul of our childhood games — he played them with us enthusiastically.

They were an extremely attractive couple. Auntie Raya, diminutive, graceful, joyous; Andrey, tall, elegant, gray-eyed. He was descended from Germans who had moved to Russia under Peter the Great and settled there. He was an art critic, a professor of fine art at Moscow University, a specialist in Renaissance art, and the head curator of the Pushkin Museum of Fine Arts. He was a remarkable storyteller who often joined my father in a wonderful yarn-spinning duet. We their children grew up to the sound of their cadences.

Despite Andrey's prestigious titles, the Gubers had a very difficult life. They lived in a huge communal apartment, in a fairly small room partitioned, like a railroad car, into compartments. Reinforcing the railroad imagery, their kids slept in bunk beds, with Shurik in the top bunk above Marishka. There was simply not enough floor space for two regular children's beds. Books took up most of the available space. Friends would insist that Andrey should try to obtain a better apartment, but he kept trying and failing, lacking the special skills required for battling or bribing bureaucrats. Eventually, an opportunity did come up to buy a small cooperative apartment, but the process of moving killed him — in sorting and packing his books, he overworked himself and had a heart attack. The doctors could not save him.

His memorial service took place in the Italian courtyard of the Pushkin museum of Fine Arts. A small orchestra played beautiful music and Pushkin's poetry was recited. It did not feel like a funeral at all and it felt as if Andrey was still here — that the statue of David by Michelangelo, the frescoes on the walls, and the chimaeras on the vaulted ceilings above us were all joining in to bid him farewell. Speakers described him as a man who would remain forever among the treasures he had so lovingly preserved during difficult times.

Such was the man who, back in 1953 during the terrible days after my Papa's arrest, sent his daughter Marishka to our house to tell me that I was to come to their home every day for dinner from then on. These daily visits carried a tremendous risk for the Gubers, all the more so because they lived in a communal apartment where any tenant could inform on them. But the Gubers knew no fear. They fed me every day and gave me food to take home to Mama. Later, the daily visits were replaced with daily meetings with their son Shurik, who would meet me in some busy Moscow street to hand me a pot of food and take back an empty pot from the day before.

I will never forget my visits to the Gubers. As I have mentioned, MGB agents were always stationed in our stairway, in the courtyard, in the street, waiting to follow Mama and me. I could easily pick them out of a crowd — it wasn't at all difficult since they all looked remarkably similar. Mama taught me how to lose them. I would go down into the subway, get into a car, and stand close to a door. As the doors were about to close, I would quickly jump out, hop on a train going in the opposite direction, and ride for two or three stations. On my way to the Gubers' home or to my rendezvous with Shurik, I would repeat the operation several times. I had to be absolutely sure I had lost them; otherwise, I was supposed to return home.

My tradecraft worked: I don't remember ever failing to lose my "tail." But going out into the street was torture, for another reason.

There were barrack-like tenements in our courtyard. Our concierge, Lucia — the one who had told me to open the door for the MGB agents who had come to arrest my father — lived there. Even before dawn on the morning after Papa's arrest, the inhabitants of the barracks had begun spreading the rumor that my father had taken pus from cancerous corpses and rubbed it into the skin of healthy people. The boys from the barracks enthusiastically took it upon themselves to avenge my father's monstrous crimes, pelting me with anything and everything they could get their hands on: rotten vegetables, dead mice and rats, and sometimes even cobblestones. No matter how humiliating it was, I had to turn tail and run; if I wasn't fast enough, I would get a beating.

4.8 *My Father's Return*

One day in February 1953, my mother returned home looking like death. They had rejected her weekly care package (one hundred rubles) for my father. "Don't bring any more, it's no longer necessary," said the MGB man on duty as he looked at his list. He refused to answer Mama's questions. There could be only one explanation: Papa was no longer alive. The days dragged on — black, empty, dark.

March 4, 1953. Stalin is very ill. Mama can't tear herself away from the radio. She listens tensely, eagerly, her breathing uneven. Mama is silent, waiting.

March 5, 1953. It is finished! The tyrant is dead! For the first time, some kind of faint, uncertain light penetrates the black night behind my mother's eyes. If only Papa were alive; so much could change now!

March 7 — or perhaps it was the 8th. The phone rings. A male voice says: "I am calling at the request of the Professor. The Professor asked me to tell you that he is healthy, he's feeling fine, and is concerned about his family. What should I tell the Professor?"

"The Professor!" Not the murderer, not the monster, not the scum of the earth, but the Professor. He is alive!

"We are fine," my mother replied, almost screaming, "tell him we are fine, we are healthy, we are… happy!" (This was hardly an appropriate word to use in those days of national mourning.)

He is alive! I fly to the Gubers' with my earth-shaking news. They embrace me, cry with me, and Aunt Raya runs to the kitchen to bake a cake. "For the wake," she tells the shocked neighbors an awkward lie, "we want to remember Joseph Vissarionovich Stalin in the Russian tradition!" I race back home with the cake and other treats for our great celebration.

Stalin lies in state in the Hall of Columns. Yet even still, his corpse thirsts for new victims: hundreds of people — sincere mourners or merely curious gawkers — are trampled to death by the disorderly crowd during the public viewing of the body. Meanwhile, we celebrate his death and my father's life, both together at our home. For the first time in my life, I feel my alienation from the surrounding Soviet reality so piercingly and acutely. I feel it no longer as a child but as a grown-up. It is the beginning of my adulthood.

Now Mama and I live on hope. Mama again sends off care packages. It turns out that Papa was moved to a special confinement unit where, among other privations, he was not allowed to receive packages. We learn later that he refused to sign false accusations against either himself or others, and his jailers transferred him to a special prison that was even better equipped than Lubyanka to persuade him otherwise. He was subjected to sleep deprivation; for about ten days they did not let him close his eyes. And even then, he didn't sign.

Days and weeks pass. No news, no news. Then, late at night on April 3, our dog Topsy suddenly goes wild. She starts running up and down the hallway, pushing against the sealed door of our dining room, then against the front door, clearing my cot in a single leap. I'm in a panic — they're coming to arrest Mama!

The telephone rings. My father's voice: "My darlings, it's me! I'll be home in a minute. I'm calling from the telephone booth downstairs. I didn't want you to faint at my sudden appearance."

Topsy sits frozen at the door; only her tail wags like a pendulum, back and forth, back and forth. She whines impatiently. A minute or two later, the doorbell rings. It's Papa! With him is an MGB colonel and the same lieutenant who took him away; now he carries Papa's little suitcase. Topsy is the first to greet him — with a record-breaking leap from the floor she throws herself at his neck, licking his lips, nose, eyes. My mother's turn is next, then mine. We laugh and cry, all at once.

The colonel says, "We return the Professor to you." While the lieutenant removes the seals from our doors, the colonel telephones somewhere: "Comrade General, the Professor has been delivered. There is much joy, many tears."

The solemn black suit pinned with the Order of Lenin drapes over my father's gaunt frame like an oversized shirt on a clothes hanger. The Order of Lenin, which he received for wartime service to the Fatherland, now dazzles our eyes. He is alive and home with a certificate of full rehabilitation, all charges against him expunged! Here it is, the certificate — we examine it, holding it up to the light, but can't seem to be able to read the words. At this moment we are having trouble comprehending anything.

The colonel says that all our confiscated property will be returned to us later that afternoon. He then wishes us luck and he and the lieutenant take their leave. The three of us are left alone. Papa, Mama, and I. Papa talks, Mama listens. I can't hear a thing they say; I just sit there looking at Papa.

Six o'clock in the morning. The radio announces to the world the end of the killer-doctor affair and the full rehabilitation of all the accused. The doorbell rings: our neighbors the Beklemyshevs come to see us, and behind them our other neighbors, the Kaplans. They've been up all night, hearing the noise coming from our apartment and thinking my mother was being arrested. But then they heard the radio announcement.

From that moment on, the door of our apartment never closed. Within a few hours, the entire building has come to visit. There are heaps of flowers. Out of the blue, my entire school class shows up. There is no longer any need to keep secrets, and those girls who knew are rewarded for their months of silence — now they can be proud to have kept it. Everyone comes, even the girl who insulted me, with a flower in her hand! One by one, each gives a flower to Papa. I am crying. (Even now I am crying as I write these lines.) Then my schoolteachers come — all of them except my history teacher. They ask me when I plan to return to school. I answer, "Tomorrow!"

Lord, what a day, what a celebration! Papa calls around to his friends who were arrested in the Doctors' Plot; all of them are back home. Not all are able to move about or even to talk yet, but all are back home.

Mama and Papa telephone my sister Lyalya. A year ago she graduated from the Second Moscow Medical School and was sent on a mandatory two-year post-graduation assignment to an outpatient clinic located in the small, old, provincial town of Toropets, about a night's train ride from Moscow. Her future husband, then a student, visited her during his winter break in January 1953 and left her pregnant. She was in her first days of pregnancy when our father was arrested. The MGB Headquarters had informed the local MGB department in Toropets that she was a daughter of a doctor-killer. During those two months that my father was incarcerated, they interrogated and beat Lyalya, cracking her lower jaw because she refused to sign a paper naming our father and her Jewish teachers at the Second Moscow Medical School as spies. She never signed it!

Two days after my father's return from prison, my parents went to Toropets and brought my sister back to Moscow. She had not completed her two-year work assignment in Toropets, but my father's reputation helped her secure an internship and residency at the Botkin clinic, one of the best in Moscow. On October 30, she delivered a dark-haired baby boy with a wide snow-white streak running from his forehead to the back of his head. At school and later at the institute, his nickname was "grayhead."

In the 1990s, my sister's family emigrated to Germany. She died in May 2017 at the age of 88.

But back to April 1953. Papa went back to his place of work, his institute. The director, Semyon Ivanovich Didenko, a remarkable man, embraced him with tears in his eyes and explained that he had tried as best as he could to hold out, but had just recently been forced to call a Party meeting that branded my father (as was routine in such cases) an enemy of the people, a murderer, a monster, and expelled him from the Party. Didenko was delighted that my father was now free, and Papa told him to forget about the meeting; he understood everything and was amazed at how long the director had managed to hold off the inevitable. When Papa returned to work, many of his colleagues couldn't look him in the eye.

Life gradually returned to normal. I went back to school. Studying was as natural to me as breathing. Soon my classmates' burning interest in me cooled and my life became easier.

And a little bit later, Lina Stern reentered our life, back from prison and exile. I became very close to her and still cherish the memories of our meetings and conversations.

April 4th became an annual celebration in our family. In the first years after Stalin's death, the survivors of the Doctors' Plot (both those who had been imprisoned and others who had waited in fear for an arrest that never came), between twenty-five and thirty people, gathered around our table on this day. Their number decreased gradually as time took its toll; none are alive today. Yet we continue to celebrate this day — the day of our rebirth.

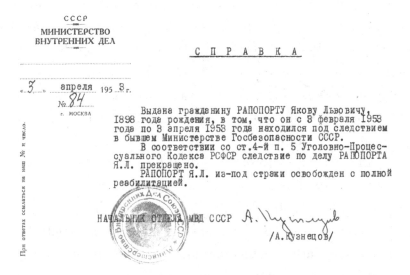

CCCP
МИНИСТЕРСТВО
ВНУТРЕННИХ ДЕЛ

С П Р А В К А

«3» апреля 195 8 г.
№ 84
г. МОСКВА

Выдана гражданину РАПОПОРТУ Якову Львовичу, 1898 года рождения, в том, что он с 3 февраля 1953 года по 3 апреля 1953 года находился под следствием в бывшем Министерстве Госбезопасности СССР.
В соответствии со ст.4-й п. 5 Уголовно-Процессуального Кодекса РСФСР следствие по делу РАПОПОРТА Я.Л. прекращено.
РАПОПОРТ Я.Л. из-под стражи освобожден с полной реабилитацией.

НАЧАЛЬНИК ОТДЕЛА МВД СССР А. Кузнецов
/А. Кузнецов/

The certificate of release from prison and complete rehabilitation issued to Yakov Rapoport by the Ministry of Foreign Affairs on April 3, 1953. From the author's archive.

5. My "Explosive" Path Toward a Career in Chemistry

In September 1952, half a year before my father's arrest, I started seventh grade, which included an introductory class in chemistry. In our first chemistry class, our teacher, Maria Moiseyevna, a dark-haired young woman with a clearly Jewish appearance, combined two colorless solutions and suddenly got a bright-red liquid. I was, as they say these days, "blown away." I was awe-struck. A world of mystery and beauty filled with wonderful possibilities opened before me. If two clear liquids could produce a red solution — what about a blue one, or a green one? I volunteered to be teacher's assistant and was allowed to set up experiments for upcoming classroom demonstrations. I set up fifteen tiny sets of Kipp's apparatus for hydrogen production in test tubes, one for each classroom desk, and when hydrogen caught fire from a lighted match with a distinctive "pop," my heart brimmed with pride for science, to which I had already decided to give my life. I put all my heart into my work and the teacher was delighted. Naïve and trusting, she began to leave me alone in the supply room where I was expected to prepare class demonstrations. I don't recall how I got my hands on a little book called *Fun Chemical Experiments and Tricks*. I practically memorized it and made an inventory of the supply room. There, in wall-mounted cupboards were treasures without number in the form of various chemicals, including many of those listed in *Fun Chemical Experiments*, and I began exploring. First, I made an innocent little "volcano" using ammonium dichromate (in plentiful supply in the cupboards), which duly erupted when I lit it with fire. I demonstrated my volcano several times in the courtyard of our apartment building, delighting my large audience.

Our building was owned by a housing cooperative set up and inhabited by medical professors, and all of us kids knew each other and got along great regardless of age or sex. Buoyed by my success and basking in their admiration, I sought new achievements. My next experiment involved nitrogen triiodide, which my book said was very unstable and in its dry form exploded easily (but safely) from the slightest movement of air. Unlike my little volcano, this experiment required me *to synthesize* the nitrogen triiodide. My first attempt at chemical synthesis was successful — the dry nitrogen triiodide detonated beautifully under my friends' feet where I had quietly spread it. Unfortunately, this trick was less popular; some of my friends got scared by the sudden popping under their feet and others got upset at me.

I had to act quickly to rehabilitate myself. That's when I read about gunpowder that could burn under water. I had everything necessary: sulphur, coal, and potassium nitrate, ready to be ground up and mixed. So I duly ground them up and mixed them together. The little book hadn't lied; what I got was gunpowder that burned very nicely under water.

Now this was a spectacle worthy of a broader audience! I started making my gunpowder in *semi-industrial* quantities... and it exploded. But how! The blast blew out the windows in the little supply room, knocked the cupboards off the walls, and broke jars of chemicals. Acids spilled out; everything swam together in one almighty mess.

The explosion brought our teachers and second-shift students running. They found me curled up under the teacher's desk in the adjoining chemistry room and my brand-new school uniform was smoldering. I was covered with glass, but thankfully, my eyes were spared. They took me to the hospital where the glass shards were removed, my burns were treated, and I was basically fine.

Unfortunately, the same could not be said of my poor teacher. She was fired, and I suspect this went on her record so she couldn't teach again. Only many years later did I understand what might have happened, not only to her but to my own family, if it hadn't been for our wonderful school principal, Vera Lukinichna Kirichenko. After all, this happened in the fall or winter of 1952, at the peak of Stalin's anti-Semitic campaign. The groundwork was being laid for the Doctors' Plot, and Dr. Vovsi and Dr. Vinogradov had been arrested. It would have been so easy to declare this explosion in a school chemistry room an intentional act of terrorism by two evil Jews, the teacher Maria Moiseyevna and her student Natalia Rapoport — both our names were unmistakably Jewish. But this didn't happen. We simply had no chemistry classes for about two months, which spanned the time needed to repair the chemistry room and recruit a new chemistry teacher. No chemistry classes for two months! My popularity with fellow students skyrocketed.

My parents were understandably very concerned about the explosion, which could have ended in tragedy. It was a miracle I hadn't been injured, disfigured, or blinded. My mother longed to see my chemistry craze pass. My father felt differently — he was glad that I was interested in science, especially one that, at least in those years, was separate and distinct from medicine. My father's greatest fear was that I might follow the family tradition and become a doctor at a time when it was notably unsafe to be a doctor *and* a Jew, a time when he himself was expecting to be arrested any day.

What my parents agreed on was the urgent need to set me straight about my "fun chemical experiments and tricks." They turned for help to our old friend Victor Kabanov, then a student in the Chemistry Department of the Moscow State University (MSU), as he was someone whom I would undoubtedly listen to. I knew Victor since my childhood. A tall, handsome boy of fourteen or fifteen, he used to be a relatively regular guest at our house. He accompanied his mother who worked with my father at the same hospital. I was ten or eleven, red-headed, freckled and funny-looking. The boy occasionally winked at me, tweaked my nose but otherwise forgot I existed. He was there to see my father, whom he loved and respected. Victor's mother worried that her good-looking son was attracting the attention of women several years older than him. My father, who was known to be well-versed in these things, tactfully imparted his experience to the boy. He enjoyed talking to him and found him very smart. When they talked, they totally forgot I was there. No one could imagine that the handsome boy would come to play a central part in my life.

Victor Kabanov graduated from high school with top marks. When I started my seventh grade, he started his first year in the

Chemistry Department of MSU. The big bang I created at school got me on Victor's radar for the first time.

As I understand it, Victor was asked by my parents to read me the riot act about chemistry being a serious science that required great care and was best left to professionals. But Victor, after asking me questions about the explosions, did not lecture me; instead, he took me to the chemistry club for high school students run by the MSU Chemistry Department, where I became a regular. I think I was the youngest there. They didn't give me any serious projects, but I watched what others were doing, entranced, and slowly learned just from being there. Victor, always busy, dropped by occasionally on his way from elsewhere, said something encouraging and ran off again.

And yet, even though I did not distinguish myself in any way at the club or at chemistry competitions between Moscow schools, the club played a decisive role in my getting into the MSU chemistry program.

I had been a straight A student and graduated high school with a gold medal, which exempted me from entrance exams and other selection formalities except for an in-person interview. I stood in the hallway with other applicants, also gold medal holders, waiting for my interview. The kids before me all came out happy after five or ten minutes. My experience was different: I was grilled in earnest for about forty-five minutes. The chemistry program had three hundred slots for each incoming class, with five or ten reserved for Jewish students under the secret quota system. Thus, for Jewish applicants, it was incredibly selective, far more than for non-Jews. I was asked questions in my interview that no mere high school student, no one without prior in-depth training in chemistry, could answer. To the surprise of my interviewers, I was able to answer them, and my name was added to the list of those admitted.

In this way, I owed my admission to MSU to Victor Kabanov; or, perhaps, ultimately, to that explosion in the chemistry room, although that is definitely not something I would recommend to anyone.

At the university, Victor took me under his wing and became my first teacher and my Master's thesis mentor. We both studied under Academician Valentin Kargin. Later, Victor became the Academician-Secretary of the Chemical Sciences Division of the Soviet Academy of Sciences; that is, the chief chemist of the country.

In those years, education was free and every college or university graduate, by way of compensation, owed the state two years of service at a job assigned to him or her by a special government commission. This first job largely determined the graduate's professional future. I graduated with distinction and Academician Kargin offered me a job at his laboratory at the Karpov Institute of Physical Chemistry in Moscow, a very nice and indeed flattering offer.

6. A Social Outcast

I got my Ph.D. at the Karpov Institute and began to build my career. I did some interesting work and had several good publications to my name when, in 1969, I suddenly became a social outcast after being caught carrying a forbidden book, Alexander Solzhenitsyn's *The First Circle*, on a tram.

That was a time of strict censorship. People were only allowed to read government-approved books, usually pulp fiction filled with lies and propaganda. Such were the only works of literature that were being published in the Soviet Union. But a separate, underground literature had emerged. Popularly known as *samizdat* ("self-published"),[5] these books were secretly reprinted often on tissue-thin paper and lent to friends, usually for one night only, so that the material could circulate widely and quickly to avoid implicating anyone as the publication and dissemination of *samizdat* carried heavy prison sentences. Reading it was also punishable, although less severely.

Solzhenitsyn's *samizdat* novel had been lent to me by my physicist friend, Ben-Tzion Tavger, a professor at the State University in the city of Gorky.

I had met Ben-Tzion by accident. After graduating from the university, I usually spent my summer vacations mountain climbing in the Crimea with my childhood friends. One day I set out alone, trying to climb up to a very beautiful place known as the "New World." I decided to take a shortcut away from the main path and soon found myself standing over a cliff. I stood on a little ledge before a narrow crevice; all I had to do was take one step forward and up, but I froze and could not get myself to take that step. I could not go back either because the ledge was not big enough for me to turn around. As often happens in those kinds of situations, I panicked. Down below me were sharp, spear-like rocks. I stood stock-still and pressed into the rock, grabbing tightly onto an outcropping, too terrified to move. With each passing second, the situation became increasingly catastrophic — my arms were numb and my knees were shaking.

Suddenly I heard men's voices in the distance, probably coming down that path, and I called for help at the top of my voice. Two men raced over to me. One of them leaned down and

---

[5] *Samizdat* refers to a book prohibited by the Soviet government that has been copied in secret on a typewriter. Up until *perestroika*, the publication and dissemination of *samizdat* was classified as a crime and carried a prison sentence.

grabbed my wrists. That was enough — my fear evaporated and I easily stepped over the crevice and reached the hard ground. What better occasion for friendship could there be? My rescuer was Ben-Tzion Tavger, a short, squat, dark-haired man with great burning, slightly bulging eyes and an Oriental appearance — even his Crimean suntan could not hide his naturally dark skin tone. I do not remember his friend's name. They were both from Gorky and also happened to be young physics professors from the Gorky State University. Ben and I became friends; he occasionally came to visit us in Moscow and we wrote letters to one another in between his visits.

In Gorky, Ben was at the heart of a circle of students who were studying Hebrew (illegally, of course) and publishing *samizdat*. Ben and his students were very good at making their *samizdat* manuscripts look like dissertations, slapping such titles on them as *A Marxist-Leninist View of the International Labor Movement*, both as camouflage and mockery. His students regularly traveled to or passed through Moscow, so Ben sent me "dissertations" for "review." I sent the books back the same way through students returning to Gorky.

Solzhenitsyn's *The First Circle* was in two "volumes." We quickly read the first volume and returned it to Gorky, but my mother was too slow in reading the second. Ben sent me an admonition: "Where is π to 2π?" (a reference to the second half of a circle). His letter arrived opened, wrinkled and ripped, but for some reason this failed to alarm me. Later we learned that by that time Ben had already been arrested, but neither I nor the student passing through Moscow on his way back to Gorky were aware of it. The student called me and asked if I had anything to send to his professor. I said I did, and we agreed to meet at the train station.

The year was 1969 and the KGB was throwing all its might into hunting political dissidents and their *samizdat*. The government was reading all my letters and listening to all my phone calls, and they noted the student's call. I was caught red-handed on the tram with the forbidden book on my way to meet him, and the student was arrested at the train station with other *samizdat* in his possession. Later I was told that his life ended tragically: he was immediately expelled from the university and drafted into the army. He had kidney disease and so he died in the army.

In 1969, the article of the criminal code dealing with *samizdat* had a provision on dissemination but none on producing the materials (this gap was later closed). In order to convict Ben under that article, the KGB needed proof that he had not only typed the books but also disseminated them. They pressed me to testify against Ben but I refused. He spent several months in jail without being charged, and then they transferred him to a psychiatric hospital (standard procedure in Soviet penal practice), kept him there a few more months and finally let him go. He moved from Gorky to Novosibirsk and then, very quickly, to Israel where he became a war hero in the 1973 Yom Kippur war before dying, still young, from a heart attack. There is a square in Israel named after Ben-Tzion Tavger.

The man who interrogated me brought me to my Institute's First Department, a local arm of the KGB. They "generously" offered me the option of resigning from my job, adding that otherwise they would fire me in some unpleasant way that might jeopardize my future employment, such as for habitual tardiness. Thankfully, I had enough presence of mind to refuse to resign. The next morning, my boss, Academician Kargin, called me into his office. "Natasha," said Kargin, "start looking for a job. I'm going to keep you here until you find one. But you're going to be demoted to technician; I can't help with that." I had an infant daughter who was often sick, so I did occasionally come to work a few seconds or minutes late. That became the official reason for downgrading me from my Ph.D. position and my salary down to a lab technician's.

I began my job search, which proved long, hard, and unsuccessful. I started by looking at decent places and even tried to get hired as a laboratory head at the Institute of Medical Polymers. They really wanted to hire me but could not due to the KGB black mark on my record. Gradually, I began setting my sights lower and eventually my husband began looking through the "help wanted" section in the *Evening Moscow* newspaper. One day, he read that the Red Rose textile factory had an opening for a tester of mechanical properties of fibers. I called them, explained that I had a Ph.D. degree and a ton of experience in their exact field, and was greeted with great enthusiasm. The next day, however, their enthusiasm had cooled... nay, had positively frozen over. I was told that the position had been eliminated...

I had hit rock bottom in my profession. It was time for cardinal change; I could not impose on Kargin's goodwill forever. For the first time, I contemplated emigration, but emigration was not an option either; this was several years before emigration from the Soviet Union officially began. The Iron Curtain extended from below the ground to above the clouds and had neither windows nor chinks. The year was 1969; Soviet tanks had just crushed the Prague Spring.

In despair, I went to see Kargin again and told him about my failure at the textile factory: "Valentin Alekseyevich, I know how difficult it is for you to keep me working here at the Karpov and I am very grateful. I've been looking non-stop all this time but no one will hire me. Yesterday, the Red Rose textile factory refused to hire me as a fiber tester. I don't know what to do but I realize that I must leave the Institute so as not to get you in trouble."

Kargin surprised me by looking at me with a mischievous gleam in his eyes and asking: "Natasha, why don't you try the Institute of Chemical Physics?" The Institute of Chemical Physics was a leading research institution of the Soviet Academy of Sciences and a dream job for any chemical scientist. I felt that one of us must surely have gone insane. "Valentin Alekseyevich, perhaps you didn't hear me. Yesterday, I was turned down by the Red Rose textile factory! How can I even think about the Institute of Chemical Physics?" "Natasha," said Kargin, "Academician Emanuel is putting together a new department at the Institute of Chemical Physics and needs people like you, with exactly your specialty. I'll talk to him." Academician Nikolay Emanuel was then the Academician-Secretary of the Chemical Sciences Division of the Soviet Academy of Sciences — that is, the chief chemist of the country (he was my friend Victor Kabanov's predecessor in that position). The next day Kargin stepped into my lab and said, "Natasha, go ahead and call Emanuel. He's ready to hire you." I felt I was in a dream and was afraid to wake up.

The next day after our conversation, Kargin flew to Italy for a week-long trip. He had to cut his trip short because his wife had fallen gravely ill back home. He rushed straight from the airport to her hospital and died of a ruptured aorta while driving home from the hospital. That was a terrible, unexpected loss and a terrible blow to me. But this I will never forget — Academician Emanuel got my phone number somehow and called me at home: "Natasha, I can understand that this is a difficult time for you, what with having lost your teacher and your whole situation. But I want to tell you that this was Valentin Alekseyevich's last request and I'm going to honor it."

Even as the chief chemist of the country, it took him several months to shepherd my appointment to the Institute of Chemical Physics through the monstrous HR (read: KGB) hurdles of the Academy of Sciences, but he did honor Kargin's request. In this way, two powerful academicians settled my human and professional fate.

I was hired for a lower-level position than my qualifications warranted, but I was elated anyway. Emanuel apologized to me for this and promised to promote me at the first opportunity. The first opportunity, however, took many years to materialize. Ten years later, I was still listed as a mere junior researcher despite the fact that my work and my publications were all on track, and I was working on my post-doctoral dissertation (a D.Sc.). All that was lacking was the correct job title and, of course, a corresponding salary. All around me, Russian (i.e., non-Jewish) guys with Communist Party memberships were passing their lower-level Ph.D. theses and being instantly promoted to senior researcher positions while I languished as a junior. This was an insult, and I finally decided to talk to the Institute's top management. The management shocked me with its frankness.

"Natasha," said the deputy director of the Institute, "this is not about you personally, everyone likes you. It's just that Academician Emanuel has set up a damn synagogue in your department and the Party district committee is unhappy with him. If he promotes you to senior researcher, he's going to have problems with the Party. Do you want Emanuel to have problems with the Party?"

I did not want Emanuel to have problems with the Party. I owed him my career. He had hired me at a critical juncture in my life when even the Red Rose textile factory had spurned me.

I asked, "So am I going to stay a junior forever? Do I have no chance for advancement?" "Why, Natasha, we're all mortal. As soon as a vacancy opens up, we'll make you senior." I could not believe my ears. "You're saying that I have to wait until one of my Jewish colleagues dies?" "Not necessarily. They don't have to die; if they retire, that will work, too."

This conversation shocked me. Once again, as with my university admission process, I was not allowed to compete fairly with my peers for professional advancement. Instead, I was being relegated to a narrow, second-class "Jewish" track. I rode the subway home and cried. I felt like I'd been flayed. I stayed home for several days, sinking into a true depression. I felt a strong desire to flee this country — to save myself, to save my daughter Victoria from ever having to participate in a similar dialog.

My husband was unprepared to countenance such drastic steps. He viewed the situation with a wise detachment worthy of a Chinese philosopher: this was the country we were living in; best to accept it and try to find the best way out of this dead end. I did not want to hear it. I fell asleep and woke up with one thing on my mind: to get out of this country! I even began to contemplate divorce, but fortunately, it did not come to that.

Gradually, the pain lessened and I became normal again. The deputy director also kept his word. When Professor Maysus, a Jewish woman in our department, passed away unexpectedly, I was immediately promoted to senior and then to leading researcher.

Around that time, I met and developed a close friendship with a wonderful couple, Irina and Yuli Daniel. Yuli was a writer while Irina was a theater artist. Yuli Daniel was one of the two named defendants in the notorious 1966 Daniel and Sinyavsky trial. They had published (abroad, under pseudonyms) books mocking the Soviet regime. Yuli spent five years in a concentration camp; Andrey Sinyavsky spent seven years. After their release, Sinyavsky emigrated to France and became a professor at the Sorbonne while Daniel stayed in Moscow. The Daniels lived in our building and I spent more time in their apartment than in my own. Yuli and Irina were a wonderful duo, and there, bathed by waves of humor, irony, and the grotesque, I exulted in this precious gift of fate. My little daughter Victoria grew up in that life-giving atmosphere and Irina mentored her as an artist.

In the Daniels' home, I came to understand something very important: freedom resides within us. I stopped feeling traumatized by the unfreedom of our exterior lives and forgot about emigration for many years.

2 Chapter   My Father Yakov Rapoport

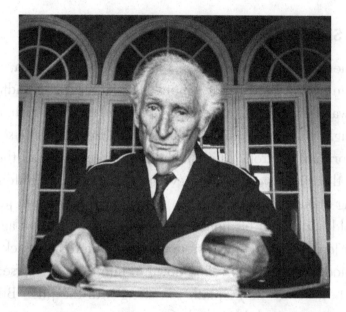

Yakov Rapoport at 91 with his manuscript *The Doctors' Plot of 1953*.

My father was born in 1898 and died in 1996. He used to joke that he was trying to get into the Guinness Book of Records as a man whose life spanned three centuries. He was just four years short of this record. The 20th century barreled across his life, doing its best to shatter, cripple, and destroy him. In truth, the one record my father certainly did set was the sheer number of things that happened to him that might easily have ended in tragedy, and yet, despite it all, he lived a happy life due to his innate wisdom and optimism, his gift of being able to see the funny side of every situation, and the steadfast support he had from my mother. A brilliant man, he loved his profession, Jewish jokes, good food and wine, his friends and beautiful women, and was very popular with everyone. He was a dazzling storyteller. Below are some episodes of my father's remarkable life.

1. The Shattered Globe

My father was born in Simferopol, the capital city of Crimea, which was then part of the Russian empire. His father (my grandfather Leib) was the director of a technical secondary school where he also taught Russian and mathematics. As it happened, the school, which primarily enrolled Jewish children, became one of the targets of the 1905 *pogrom* (anti-Jewish mob attack) in Simferopol. Hearing about the pogrom at the school, my father, then just six years old, ran out of his house and headed there. At that age, he did not look Jewish. He was stopped by a mounted Cossack waving a bloody sword, who yelled down to him from his horse: "Go home, boy, before they squash you along with the Jids!" But my father ran on toward the school anyway.

During the pogrom, my grandfather had been beaten half to death; he was unconscious and barely breathing. A special team that was collecting the victims of the *pogrom* thought him dead and took him to the morgue, where they dumped him among the corpses. After the *pogrom* was over, a neighbor of his went to the morgue with a handcart to find and take back her family members. Hearing a moan from underneath a pile of bodies, she dug around and found my grandfather, severely injured but alive. She wheeled him home in her cart and my grandmother nursed him back to life.

Soon after recovering from his injuries, my grandfather left his family for a young Tatar woman. He had two kids with her, in addition to the three kids he had with my grandmother. In 1922, he and his Tatar girlfriend were found stabbed to death in their home, supposedly by burglars. Somebody informed my father of the tragedy but when he arrived there, the house was empty. The fate of the kids remains unknown.

My grandmother outlived her estranged husband by twenty years and was shot by the Nazis in 1942, together with her elder son and other Crimean Jews. Regrettably, I have never met any of my grandparents from either side. They had died before I was born or perished in the Holocaust.

...When my father got to the school during the *pogrom*, my grandfather was no longer there. Everything was smashed, broken, defiled. A crushed blue globe lay on the floor among shattered glass and broken furniture. For my father, this caved-in model of the Earth became a symbol of Jewish *pogroms*. He was destined to live through several of them during his long life.

2. His Stormy Path to Profession in Medicine

In 1915, my father graduated from high school with honors and went from Simferopol to St. Petersburg to continue his studies. He first enrolled at the Musical Conservatory, where the famous Russian composer Alexander Glazunov examined him and was very impressed.

At the same time, having somehow procured a duplicate set of papers, my father took the entrance examination for the Medical Institute and was also accepted. After thinking about it for a while, he chose medicine over music.

Lacking the residency papers that were required at the time for Jews to live in St. Petersburg, he rented a corner from a hotel doorman who exploited him shamelessly, taking advantage of his undocumented status.

In 1917, there was a typhus epidemic in Russia. My father contracted typhus and spent twenty-four days in the hospital. He pulled through by a miracle. Having barely recovered, he was issued a rifle and a revolver and, together with his fellow students, was sent to guard the members of the Provisional Government (formed by members of the Russian parliamentary assembly, the State Duma, to take over from the failing monarchy). But then the October Revolution began and the Bolsheviks seized power. Some of the members of the State Duma hid in the hospital disguised as patients, but rebel sailors found them and smothered them to death with hospital pillows. That's when my father threw his rifle into the Neva river, rigged a false bottom in his suitcase for his revolver and decided to go back to Simferopol to rejoin the Medical Institute, which had relocated there and was staffed with excellent professors from St. Petersburg.

The way to Crimea passes through Ukraine, which was then under the control of the Hetman (chieftain) Skoropadsky, having broken off from Russia in the revolutionary turmoil. Trains originating in Russia stopped on the Russian side of the Ukrainian border, while trains bound for Crimea started from the Ukrainian side. The distance between the last station on the Russian line and the first station on the Ukrainian line had to be covered by horse cab. This immediately gave rise to a new form of business: cab drivers sometimes assembled a group of passengers and robbed them along the way, killing those who tried to resist. Word spread quickly and people began to look for others to travel with, trying to join groups where at least one person was armed.

My father was armed. He safely reached his home in Simferopol and continued his medical studies. Crimea was then in the hands of the Whites[1] under Baron Wrangel and my father worked as a medic (*Feldscher*) at their hospital. Then the Whites drafted him and sent him to the frontlines, but he never got there because the Red guerrillas had pushed the Whites back in the meantime. Reds put up notices everywhere demanding that all persons who had collaborated with Baron Wrangel hand in their weapons and come in to be registered. Working at the hospital was considered collaboration.

The young medics gathered in secret to discuss the situation. Their opinions were divided. Some believed that in the civilized world, hospital work was not considered treasonable regardless of who controlled the hospital, and therefore the medics at a White hospital should have nothing to fear from the Reds. Thanks to his St. Petersburg experience, my father had a better understanding of the Bolsheviks and said they should flee immediately. As a result, the group split in two — the more trusting souls remained in Simferopol and showed up to be registered while the rest fled into the Crimean mountains to make their way back to Russia. Everyone who stayed in town and registered was shot.

My father shuttled between his home and the mountains, carrying food and medications back to his group. Once, in 1921, when my father was at home, the ChK (the predecessor of the NKVD, the MGB, the KGB, and today's FSB) came to search the house. My grandmother, seeing them out in the street, called out to my father: "Run!" He jumped out the back window and managed to escape. He spent a few days with his friends, who helped him obtain false documents in the name of one Ionka Filker, a

---

[1] The *White Guard* or the *Whites* was a loose confederation of Anti-Communist forces that fought the Bolsheviks, also known as the *Reds*.

student at a weavers' technical school. Using these documents, my father went to Moscow.

A former student at my grandfather's school, now a lawyer, lived in Moscow. He tried to tell my father: "You should continue as Ionka Filker! A weaver is a nice profession, and your papers are great!" But my father disagreed; he wanted to be a doctor, not a weaver, and he was quite fond of his own last name, Rapoport.

He tried to enroll at the Medical Institute in Moscow, hoping to have his prior attendance at the Medical Institute in St. Petersburg credited to him, but all those records had been lost. It took tremendous effort to convince the Moscow program to admit him to the fifth year on probation. A month later, he was their best student, but in order to graduate, he would have to retake all of the exams for the preceding four and a half years... And then a miracle happened. A friend of my father's called and said that his wife had arrived from Simferopol and brought my father's real papers, which my grandmother had found. My father's student transcript was among them. This was all the more miraculous because the train his friend's wife was riding had been stopped by bandits who robbed all the passengers, leaving her only the bundle containing my father's papers!

That same year, my father graduated from the Moscow University School of Medicine with a degree in pathology.

3. The Actor of an "Anatomical Theater" and Correspondence with Christiaan Barnard

"I, too, am an actor. An actor in an *anatomical* theater, to be precise." That is how my father once introduced himself to an actual theater actor.

My father, a pathologist, got all his work from attending physicians, whom he jokingly called his "employers." Their failures, errors or mishaps were what ultimately brought their patients to the pathology department. As a pathologist, my father had the last word on what had gone wrong with each case. The doctors admired him. He was their oracle, their final arbiter, and yet he explained their mistakes to them with extreme gentleness, without injuring their professional pride. At the regular hospital conferences where causes of patients' deaths were analyzed, he would never accuse or reproach a physician but rather explain the cause of the patient's death in a way that showed deep respect for the doctor's work. However, he was merciless toward professional ignorance or incompetence. I have heard many generations of doctors say that they counted it as their great professional fortune to have been able to learn from my father or work with him.

My father's name as a pathologist became well known to medical professionals around the globe.

In 1966, he was elected chairman of the International Congress of Pathology, which was to be held in Venice, Italy. We knew all the details of his upcoming trip down to the smallest minutia, but in those years, there was an unofficial travel ban on Jews and the Soviet Foreign Ministry never got around to issuing him a passport... His chair at the Congress, marked with a little Soviet flag, stood vacant. The colleague who replaced him did not take his chair.

One memorable episode of my father's illustrious medical career was associated with a letter he got from Dr. Chris Barnard. On December 3, 1967, in Cape Town, South Africa, Dr. Chris Barnard performed the first ever human-to-human heart transplant. Dr. Barnard's first patient, Louis Vashkansky, received the heart of a young woman by the name of Denise Darvall, who had been declared brain dead following a road accident. Mr. Vashkan-sky survived the surgery but died 18 days later from pneumonia. A month after his first operation, on January 2, 1968, Dr. Barnard transplanted another heart to his second patient, 59-year old Philip Blaiberg. Mr. Blaiberg received the heart from a 24-year-old man, Clive Haupt, who had collapsed on a Cape Town beach the day before. This surgery was considered successful; Mr. Blaiberg lived for 19 months and 15 days after the surgery before dying from heart complications in August of 1969. In the following seven years, Dr. Barnard performed ten more heart or heart-and-lung surgeries. Two of his patients became long-term survivors. Barnard's experiments were considered a remarkable success.

Seeking my father's opinion, Dr. Barnard sent him the tissue slides from the original and transplanted hearts of his first two patients, Vashkansky and Blaiberg. In both cases, the patients obtained their new hearts from young donors. Dr. Barnard was interested in the changes that occurred in the transplanted hearts, especially that of Mr. Blaiberg, who lived with his donor heart for a year and a half. My father found that over that period, his new heart, obtained from a 24-years old donor, underwent the same changes that were present in his own 59-years old heart before its removal and which had brought him to the operating table in the first place. Based on this finding, my father formulated conditions under which heart transplants would be advantageous, in contrast to other situations where the transplants would not be favorable. Dr. Barnard responded with a very warm letter of gratitude.

4. Our Family

In 1924, a year after graduation, my father married my mother. He was a young professor of pathology while my mother was a new graduate from the same university with a degree in physiology. A family legend claims that my father married my mother, Sophya (Sonya) Epstein, by mistake. Dad's friends wanted to introduce him at the graduation party to a pretty graduate by the name of Betty Epstein. At the party, my father saw my future mom dancing and liked her. He asked his neighbor who she was and was told her last name: Epstein. Dad was overjoyed and fell in love on the spot. He found an opportunity to ask my mother to dance and kept her to himself all evening. His friends noticed his mistake and said, "Yakov, this is not the right Epstein! You want Betty, and this is Sonya!" But it was too late. My father declared that he wanted *this very* Epstein, and soon they were married. Betty occasionally came to visit our family later and always jokingly lamented my father's "mistake."

My parents' first quarter century together was very difficult. They lived in Soviet "communal apartments" crammed with people, with one family to a room. In addition, Aunt Rosa came to live with them. My parents joked that my mother brought her into the marriage as her "dowry."

Aunt Rosa used to be the director of my mother's school in the city of Vitebsk before the Revolution. She spent half of her life in Paris and taught French in school. In the chaos of the October Revolution, she lost her mind and tried to kill herself. My mother, a paragon of kindness and compassion, took her in, and Aunt Rosa lived with our family up till her death. Until my parents got their own apartment, thirty years after their wedding day, she shared their room in the communal apartment; her bed was separated from my newlywed parents' bed by a thin makeshift screen. My father found her company depressing but he was patient and tried to lighten the gloom by making jokes. For as long as I can remember, Aunt Rosa always grumbled, moaned and complained that she was dying, but my father joked that she had forgotten how to actually do it. After I was born, Aunt Rosa spoke only French to me. As such, I became bilingual in my childhood. Aunt Rosa died at the end of the 1940s, at the age of almost a hundred. After her death, I quickly forgot all my French.

Our pre-war apartment building had been destroyed by the German bomb, and after the war we got a room in a different communal apartment. This apartment housed seven families, including ours. It had only one toilet and one separate bathroom. Everyone had to be at work at the same time, so there was a morning schedule to use the toilet. Using it when nature called outside of one's allotted time slot sparked tremendous fights. A strict schedule was also set up that dictated each family's precise day of the week and time of day to take a bath or shower.

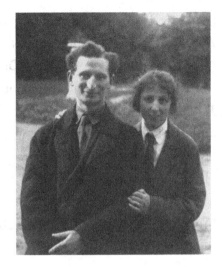

Yakov and Sophya Rapoport newlyweds, 1924.

At 25 square meters (270 square feet), our room in that apartment was fairly large by the standards of the time and my father partitioned it to create a tiny separate room for me and my mother. The remaining space, which we called the big room, served as dining room, living room, my parents' study, and my father's bedroom all at once. During the day, I did my homework in it.

My mother's cousin, Aunt Anna Yakhnina, also sometimes stayed with us. I loved her very much. In her youth, Aunt Anna had openly spoken out against the Bolsheviks. The fact that she survived the Great Purges and the later repressions was nothing short of a miracle. She was an epidemiologist; she dealt with the outbreaks of typhus and cholera. For the contribution she made to public health by combating the epidemics of infectious diseases, she was granted the honor of burial at the prestigious Novodevichye cemetery.

In the late 1940s, Stalin green-lighted the construction of cooperative housing and the professors of medicine set up a cooperative society called "Medic." In 1951, we moved from the communal apartment into our own, four-room apartment my parents had purchased.

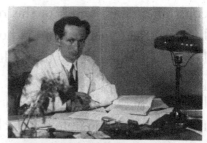
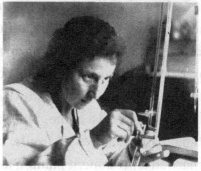

My father and mother at work. Late 1930s.

It was an unbelievable luxury! For the first time in their 27 years of marriage, my parents had their own separate bedroom!

Life in such incredibly cramped conditions as those that existed in communal apartments was not conducive to marital happiness. But my parents, besides physical love, were also united in deep friendship and their marriage was very strong until my mother's death, despite numerous romantic campaigns waged against my father by much younger women.

Unsurprisingly, my father was very popular with women. When a pretty woman came into view, his eyes would take on a special gleam and he would erupt into fireworks of wit and charm. The ladies were drawn to this flame and, like moths, got their wings singed because my father was an old-school Jewish family man who treasured my mother. She loved him selflessly, guarding his rest and sleep, trying to bring him joy and never putting any constraints upon him. For this reason, my father felt comfortable bringing his female admirers home to dinner, to show them that he had a great family and they had no hope. Of course, the ladies persevered. Among them were all kinds: some were nice, others less so. Not-so-nice ladies tended to disappear fairly quickly; my father had a strong defense mechanism and good taste.

Occasionally, things got more serious. One of my father's admirers was dazzlingly beautiful, with sharply angled black brows over blue eyes and an amazing figure, although with a shrewish personality. She was mortally bored with her own husband, a professor, and was on the prowl for a replacement, someone with both money and a name. She chose my father and mounted a sustained attack across all fronts, but my father held firm. Later, she married a prominent painter, a member of the Soviet Academy of Fine Arts.

But he did have his flings, some of them lasting a while. A colleague of my mother who nourished fond hopes regarding her once tried telling her that he had seen my father at the theater with another woman several times.

"I don't care how Yakov L'vovich feels about other women. I care how he feels about me!" said my mother, cutting her suitor off and curing him forever of any desire to tell tales, as well as all his hopes.

In my childhood and teen years, the mating dance taking place around my father really annoyed me. I could not understand what all these ladies saw in him. To me, he was not handsome: of middling height, with a too-high forehead and an aquiline beak of a nose. I shuddered when people told me I looked like my father. I pitched fits, blaming my mother, in all seriousness, for having had me with such an ugly man. My mother was saddened and tried to convince me otherwise, but to no avail, especially because in my youth I was terribly unlucky in love. I was a late bloomer, a gawky, freckled redhead, and boys refused to take me seriously.

And the worst was that my father's appearance never seemed to hinder him. His popularity with women both intrigued and annoyed me. I was too naïve to understand the impact of his irresistible charm and sparkling wit. These things, to me, were a given; they were simply a part of our lifestyle.

Later, when I grew up and became wiser, a new problem emerged: my father became that yardstick I used to measure my own suitors. Few of them could have any hope of measuring up. I was, however, fortunate to meet my husband Volodya. My father and mother loved him. In those days of housing shortages, when parents, children and grandchildren spent their whole lives living all cramped together, interpersonal tensions could turn family life into living hell. Fortunately, my parents always enjoyed Volodya's company and there were never any tensions between them despite dwelling together.

My mother died in 1971 of an internal hemorrhage which, as sometimes happens in medical families, was not recognized in time. My father's "ladies" saw their chance in her death. Before I could blink, one of my own girlfriends almost became my father's girlfriend. She was young, temperamental, and not yet forty, while my father was over seventy. I was horrified to realize what she was after. I doubt that my father would have lasted a year with her.

Katya saved the day. She and my father met at the cemetery. Katya's husband had passed away a year before my mother. He was an air force general, decorated for his service in the battle for Stalingrad. He was buried next to my mother, in the next enclosure. My father regularly visited my mother's grave and often saw a sweet, elegant woman who was visiting a nearby grave. She looked much younger than her sixty years. That is how their romance began and it continued for twenty-five years until my father's death. He was genuinely in love, bouncing around with joy like a boy despite his seventy-three years. At first, I was very jealous for my mother's sake — she had lived through the darkest years of my father's life while Katya got his best and happiest years. But Katya was very devoted to my father and brightened his old age, so I came to love her dearly.

5. Our Family Friends and Lev Landau

My parents' integrity, dignity, and my father's famous sense of humor attracted brilliant people of my parents' generation to our house. They were prominent intellectuals — leading scientists, artists, actors, writers, musicians; you name it. The Head of the Pushkin Museum of Fine Arts, Andrey Guber; a physicist, Lev Landau; a physiologist, Lina Stern; an artist, Robert Falk; a test pilot, Nikolai Ribko; a pianist, Maria Yudina; an actor and stage director, Solomon Mikhoels; etc, etc.

As a pathologist, my father sometimes had to perform autopsies on his friends when they passed away. He used to say that this was his way of paying his last respects to a friend. It was very hard on him.

One of those friends was a world-famous physicist and Nobel Prize laureate, Lev Landau (friends and colleagues called him Dau). He was awarded the Nobel Prize in 1962 for his pioneering theories. My father and Dau met through Elena Berezovskaya, the wife of Dau's closest associate, Yevgeny Lifshitz. For many years, Berezovskaya worked at my father's lab.

Landau and Lifshitz and their families shared a two-story, five-room apartment provided to them by another Nobel Prize laureate in physics, Pyotr Kapitsa, the director of the Institute of

Physical Problems where they both worked. Dau's family occupied the three rooms on the upper floor while Lifshitz lived on the lower floor. They often had very intense scientific discussions and also complemented each other, forming a productive team in which Landau's brilliant scientific ideas were clearly conveyed by Lifshitz. They co-authored the ten-volume *Course of Theoretical Physics*, a seminal textbook used by many generations of theoretical physicists all over the world. It has been said of these works that not a single word had been written by Dau and not a single thought could be attributed to Lifshitz.

Dau's relatively short life was extraordinarily eventful, crammed full of fortunate or tragic incidents that followed one after another at breakneck speed. At the age of twenty-one, Dau was awarded a Rockefeller fellowship that allowed him to spend two years at various physics institutes across Europe. He worked mostly in Copenhagen under one of the greatest physicists of the twentieth century, Niels Bohr (winner of the 1922 Nobel Prize in physics). During his years as a Rockefeller fellow, Dau visited the Ernest Rutherford laboratory where he met Pyotr Kapitsa, who spent over ten years working with Rutherford at Cambridge. In 1934, Kapitsa went back to Russia for what was supposed to be a short visit, but the Soviet authorities prevented him from returning to England. Stuck in Moscow, Kapitsa founded the Institute of Physical Problems.

The encounter with Kapitsa was Dau's lucky star. It would not be an exaggeration to say that when the time came, it was Kapitsa who saved Dau's life. In April 1938, during Stalin's purges, Dau was arrested by the NKVD, taken to Lubyanka prison and threatened with transfer to the even more terrible Lefortovo prison. There is no doubt that Dau would have been executed or died in prison. He was saved by a stroke of luck. A year after Dau's arrest, in April 1939, the NKVD chief Nikolay Yezhov was himself arrested and replaced with Lavrenty Beria. The resulting period of power transition was a relatively quiescent time compared to the Great Terror of 1937. At some risk to his own life, Kapitsa decided to take a chance and wrote a letter to Vyacheslav Molotov, then Prime Minister, saying that he had just made an important discovery "in the most puzzling field of modern physics" and that the only theoretician who could explain his discovery was the currently incarcerated physicist Lev Landau. A month later, after a year of imprisonment, Landau was let out of prison. Within a few months, he did, in fact, explain Kapitsa's discovery of superfluidity, which would earn both of them a Nobel Prize a few decades later. Kapitsa admired Landau's extraordinary brilliance and invited Landau and Lifshitz to work at his institute.

Dau and his wife Kora sometimes visited us, and we in turn visited them too. He was strikingly handsome and brilliant, and I remember him very well from my teens and early twenties. Like my father, Dau had a wonderful sense of humor. Whenever the two of them met, bursts of laughter could be heard from a long distance away. Some of their jokes were off-color and my mother would glare at them to remind them of my presence at the table. That never stopped them. Now I regret that I neither understood nor remembered their conversations and jokes.

I will refrain from discussing the details of Dau's personal life, which I knew through overhearing private conversations between my parents. But I can state here what is well known to everyone who knew Dau: he was an ardent proponent of free love and tried to impose this attitude on his friends and students. With my father, he failed. I am not calling my father a saint by any means, but family always came first for him.

On January 7, 1962, Dau was severely injured in a car accident on his way from Moscow to the town of Dubna, about 125 km (78 mi) from Moscow, which served as a base for highly advanced research in physics. There were four people in the car. Landau, who sat in the back, was the only one who got injured. Ironically, even the box of eggs they were carrying to Dubna remained intact.

Dau's traumas were virtually incompatible with life. He remained in a coma for a month and a half. My father was actively involved in coordinating medical care for his friend, contacting foreign colleagues with requests to provide badly needed medications and prostheses. Our apartment became one of the headquarters of that campaign. My assignment was to respond to telephone calls from France. My fluent French was long gone; I could barely manage, and my dad was very impatient and angry with me.

Dau survived the accident but was never again his old brilliant self. He died six years later from the complications of his injuries. As a gesture of last respect to his friend, my father performed an autopsy on Dau. It was extremely hard on him; he came back home very depressed and said, "All these years Dau was in terrible pain, probably unbearable, and everyone thought he was just being fussy."

My father found Landau's brain to be unusual in size and structure and took a lot of photographs. He did not dissect Dau's brain but took it out intact and passed it on to the Moscow Brain Institute for study.

Let me say a few words about that institution and the scientists that created it. Collections of preserved brains of great thinkers exist in many countries. The idea of creating a "Brain Pantheon" in the Soviet Union was put forward in 1927 by the great neurologist and psychiatrist Vladimir Bekhterev, with the major goal being to show to the world the superiority of Soviet minds. In Bekhterev's vision, the Brain Pantheon would exhibit the brains of Soviet celebrities and exceptional individuals recognized as geniuses — scientists, artists, musicians, actors, and politicians.

However, Bekhterev's life was cut short. On December 23, 1927, he was invited to the Kremlin as a neurologist to perform a medical examination on Stalin, whom he incautiously diagnosed as paranoid. That night, Bekhterev and his wife were invited to attend the ballet *Swan Lake* at the Bolshoi Theater. During the intermission, he ate two portions of ice cream. According to some sources, after the show, the Director of the Bolshoi Theater invited him for a cup of tea in his office. Bekhterev sickened suddenly and died of food poisoning the same night. His own brain was removed for future study, but no actual autopsy was performed and the body was hastily cremated. There is little doubt that Bekhterev's tragic death was the result of Stalin's revenge for a diagnosis he did not like.

After Bekhterev's death, his idea of creating a Brain Pantheon in Moscow was realized by the world's leading expert on brain architecture, German neuroscientist Oskar Vogt. Bekhterev's own brain was sectioned and examined in Vogt's lab. In 1928, Vogt's lab became the Moscow Brain Institute. Brain specimens of geniuses, as well as those of average people, were collected there for comparison.

One of the goals of the newly formed institution was to further enhance the canonization of Lenin, the Great Leader of the October Revolution and the founder of the Soviet Union. The Communist Party was vigorously indoctrinating Soviet citizens with the idea that Lenin was an "all-time genius." Lenin's body was embalmed and exhibited in the Mausoleum that was built in the heart of the country — Moscow's Red Square. The prevailing wisdom then was that the size and architecture of the brain was evidence of the intellectual ability of its owner. Lenin's brain was studied by Professor Vogt himself. But his results sparked an incredible controversy: rather than being gigantic and oversized, Lenin's brain turned out to be smaller than average! After several years of study, Vogt finally announced that, nevertheless, some areas in Lenin's cerebral cortex appeared to be unusually well developed, suggesting quick decision making. To avoid further embarrassment, the brains collected in the Brain Pantheon were locked away and no longer open for public viewing.

6. Medical Anecdotes and My Father's Legendary Sense of Humor

No matter how hard, scary, and unpredictable life was in the USSR, it was still life. People were falling in love, dating, marrying, and bringing up kids. Friendship and a sense of humor helped us to survive in a precarious environment.

When I was a child, I committed some of my father's stories to memory so that I could understand them when I was old enough.

There was one time I remember Papa making fun of the bureaucrats in Human Resources who were faced with a dilemma. The year was 1948 and Stalin's vicious anti-Semitic campaign had just begun with massive firings, arrests, and executions of Jewish intellectuals. The HR stooges at the Second Moscow Medical School were being pressured from above to fire the director of the school, a man with the distinctly Jewish name of Abraham Borisovich Topchan. The director was well-liked by everyone at the school, both professors and students, and for a long time the bureaucrats could not find an appropriate excuse. At last, having failed to come up with anything, they simply announced, "Topchan, Abraham Borisovich, is dismissed."

"What idiots," my father scoffed. "They should have just said: 'Topchan, being Abraham Borisovich, is dismissed.'" Papa's friends laughed, but I felt that it was not happy laughter. At that time, Jewish intellectuals no longer had any reason to laugh…

When I grew up, the night life of my generation usually took place in the cramped kitchens of our apartments. They were castles that shielded us from the oppressive absurdity of the official Soviet life. The social mores of the Moscow intelligentsia were very different from those of its American counterparts. No one ever thought of calling ahead and asking if they could drop by next Friday from 7 to 9 pm. People could and did show up unannounced. If they called at all, it was to say that they were heading over, and sometimes they just showed up. The hosts were always glad to see their friends.

Big groups used to gather in these tiny kitchens, crowded but happy. We drank vodka and ate whatever was available, told jokes and stories, and shared our news. My father liked to participate in our gatherings and my friends adored him. He was a brilliant man, known not only for his professional skills in pathology but also for his sparkling wit. Perhaps he tried to compensate for the grimness of his profession by telling funny stories and jokes. These were known throughout Moscow and I am happy to share some of them with you.

6.1 *The Death Sentence*

> "Where are you taking me?"
> "To the morgue."
> "But I'm not dead yet!"
> "That's OK, we're not there yet!"
>
> A Russian joke

Austria, early 20th century. A famous Vienna doctor says to his patient: "I regret to inform you that it is time for you to put your affairs in order. You have two months left to live… Maybe two and a half. I am very sorry, but the medical science is powerless in your case."

Five years later, the doctor meets his patient in the street. He is shocked:

"It's you? You're alive?"

"Yes, doctor! After you gave me that death sentence, I went to see your colleague, Dr. X. He helped me, and now I feel great."

"What did he prescribe?"

"Thus-and-such."

"But that was the wrong treatment!"

6.2 *A Diagnosis*

Before the Russian October Revolution of 1917, there used to be a big bookstore at the very heart of Moscow on Tverskaya street called Tseytlin's. And there was also a fashionable clinic for nervous disorders run by Professor Lazar Minor. As it was considered trendy to be treated by Professor Minor, society wives all developed nervous ailments, went around sniffing smelling salts, and traveled abroad to take the waters. Mr. Tseytlin's wife kept up with the others.

One day, Professor Minor said to her: "You need to complete a course of thermal bath therapy in Baden-Baden. I will give you a copy of your patient chart in a sealed envelope, you will give it to my colleague in Baden-Baden, Professor Oppenheim, and he will take care of you."

Madame Tseytlin received her sealed envelope in August 1914 but never made it to Baden-Baden because of WWI. In 1917, the Bolsheviks took over and Tseytlin's bookstore was nationalized by the Soviets. Instead of going to Baden-Baden, Madame Tseytlin moved into a communal apartment, which she shared with my parents. And here's an interesting medical phenomenon: after the October Revolution, Madame Tseytlin never had another nervous ailment!

The Tseytlins lived next door to my parents for a few years before moving out.

One day, my father was walking down Tverskaya street, and Mr. Tseytlin was walking toward him on the other side of the street. He saw my father and dashed across the street, dodging a horsecar and yelling: "All doctors are crooks and scoundrels! I have a document, such an incredible document; I'm taking it to the Pravda newspaper tomorrow!"

It turned out that Tseytlin had been going through his papers and had found the sealed envelope given to his wife years earlier by Professor Minor. He was curious to learn about the nature of those nervous ailments that had afflicted his wife before the Revolution. He opened the envelope and found a blank piece of cardboard with a little note attached to it: "My dear Oppenheim! I am sending you my patient, Madame Tseytlin. The Tseytlins own a big bookstore in the center of Moscow." "What's the trouble, Mr. Tseytlin?" said my father, amused. "This is the most accurate diagnosis I have ever seen in my entire medical practice! Besides, I would advise you against going to Pravda. Reminding the Soviet authorities that you used to own a big bookstore in the center of Moscow could be hazardous to your and your wife's health…"

6.3 *A Foreign Trip*

Despite his international reputation, my father was not allowed to travel outside the USSR. But then someone must have gotten sloppy — in the late 1960s, he was allowed to attend the International Congress of Pathology in Prague. This was his only foreign trip. The Soviet delegation was housed in a third-rate hotel, where my father had to share a room with Professor Fogelson. There was only one bed in the room, albeit a wide one. Two senior Soviet professors, both over seventy years old, sleeping in the same bed...

At breakfast the next morning, my father said to Professor Fogelson in front of everyone: "After last night, honor demands that I marry you. When we return to Moscow, I will ask your parents for your hand in marriage."

Their colleagues, the other members of the delegation, were very much amused, and the story spread widely in their circles.

6.4 *The Old Believer: A War Story*

During WWII, my father served as chief pathologist of the North front. He had collected a massive amount of material on wartime pathology, but because photographic film was scarce, he could not preserve it on microfilms. Unable to photograph his material, my father went looking for an artist who could paint it. Someone told him that there was an exiled Old Believer (member of a proscribed Russian Orthodox sect) living in a neighboring village who used to paint icons for the local church. My father brought him to his mobile mortuary unit and sat him down at the microscope. We still have the tissue slides painted on glass by the icon painter. My father treasured these slides. He showed them at one of his birthday celebrations: "And now, let me show you what a true believer can do when he looks into a microscope!"

7. Gloria Mundi

I would like to end this chapter on my father with the following incident that occurred during my and my daughter's first trip to the West in 1989.

Victoria and I were down in the London Tube waiting for a train, which was long in coming. We were alone on the platform except for a tall black man in his late thirties or early forties who stood a short distance away from us. He kept looking over at us and I felt a bit uneasy. We talked quietly. At some point I got a feeling that he understood our conversation because he smiled when I said something funny. Finally he came by, looked at me, extended his hand... and said in Russian (with a heavy Ukrainian accent):

"Hello! I heard you speaking Russian. Are you from Russia?"

I was stunned.

"Yes, we're from Moscow, and where are *you* from? How come you speak Russian? And why do you have a Ukrainian accent?"

"I did my residency in Kiev. I am a doctor, a pathologist."

"A pathologist! What a coincidence! My father — her grandfather — is also a pathologist. He even wrote a textbook on anatomic pathology."

"Not Dr. Rapoport, by chance?"

That was incredible. A black man in the London Tube who knew my father's name!

"Yes, he is Dr. Rapoport."

"Is that right? You're the daughter of *the* Dr. Rapoport? I can't believe it! This is such an honor for me! Who would have thought that I would meet the daughter of Dr. Rapoport himself, in London! The whole world knows Rapoport's classification of immune cells, and here I am standing here and talking to his daughter! May I invite you to a pub?"

Now *that's* what true world renown looks like.

3 The Manuscript

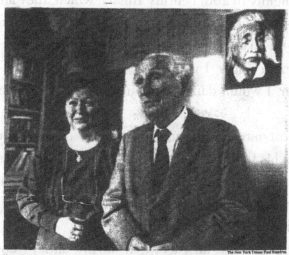

"All the News That's Fit to Print"

The New York Times

VOL.CXXXVII ... No. 47,504   *Copyright © 1988 The New York Times*   NEW YORK, FRIDAY, MAY 13, 1988   30 CENTS

New York: Today, warmer, chance late thundershower. High 85 near inland. Tonight, clearing. Low 4. Tomorrow, sunny. High 84-88. Yesterday: High 74, low 51. Details, page 1

Yakov Rapoport and his daughter, Natalya, at their home in Moscow. A portrait of Einstein adorns a wall.

The New York Times/Paul Hosefros

Soviet Survivor Relives 'Doctors' Plot'

By FELICITY BARRINGER
Special to The New York Times

MOSCOW, May 10 — To wait was Yakov Rapoport's way, and his only weapon. His memory wound itself protectively around the days in early 1953 that took him from the top ranks of Soviet medicine to a prison cell and back. When he returned, he kept silent, he kept waiting, and he kept remembering.

He remembered the throb of manacled wrists and the interrogator's words: "plotter," "poison," and "Jewish bourgeois nationalist." He remembered daydreaming that the ordeal would end in exile — "a typical paradox of Stalin's epoch, that criminals' fondest dream was choosing the

punishments for their uncommitted crimes."

After 20 years, he wrote it down. Then he waited another decade. "Now," he said in a recent interview, "the waiting is over."

On the eve of his 90th birthday, his memoirs have been published, a firsthand account of the convulsive moment of anti-Semitism called "the doctors' plot."

In April 1953, a month after Stalin's death, his successors repudiated the charges and freed the doctors. But for three decades and more afterward, the plot was never publicly put in con-

text as the culmination of five years of increasingly vicious official discrimination against Jews.

This year, that difficult confrontation has slowly begun, spurred by a reference to the doctors' plot in Mikhail S. Gorbachev's speech on Soviet history last fall. Dr. Rapoport's memoirs were accepted by the monthly magazine Druzhba Narodov, his daughter Natalya's were accepted by the monthly Yunost, and both were published in the April editions.

"Bit by bit, I've been left alone, the last of those arrested, or at least I think so," Dr. Rapoport said. "The generations that follow must know about this."

"I had to write this down to rid myself of it," said Natalya, who was 14 when she opened the apartment door

Continued on Page A8, Column 1

After the Doctors' Plot, my father lived a long life and celebrated many major birthdays. Because of his professional stature, the entire Russian medical world celebrated his jubilees with him. These public celebrations seemed to come one right after another: his 70th, 75th, 80th, 85th, 90th and so forth...

His 70th birthday was in 1968 after the end of Khrushchev's "thaw." My father stepped out on the flower-strewn stage of the Medical Institute. The audience gave him a long standing ovation, showing their admiration of the man who had managed to preserve his human dignity in 20th century Russia, which, they all felt, was in itself an act of heroism. Deeply touched, my father said, "You are treating me like an opera singer or a movie star. Except that if I were an opera singer, I would sing for you now, and if I were a ballet dancer, I would dance for you. But what can a pathologist do for you?"

The most memorable and meaningful of my father's celebrations was his 90th birthday. We, his family, barely got in. The Medic Club on Hertzen street was surrounded by a dense crowd that blocked the entrances and spilled across the street onto the opposite sidewalk.

This was because an excerpt from my father's book about Stalin's Doctors' Plot had been published by the *Druzhba Narodov* (*Friendship of Peoples*) magazine just a few months earlier, in April 1988, to mark the 35th anniversary of the release of the arrested doctors. Simultaneously, the popular magazine *Yunost* (*Youth*) published my own account of the events of the Doctors' Plot. In those information-starved days, my father's book was the first eyewitness account by a victim of those events, the first open description of the regime's official policy of anti-Semitism that had come so close to producing a Soviet version of the "final solution to the Jewish question" back in 1953. For thirty-five years, the sinister events of the Doctors' Plot had been censored out of Russian history. Our twin publications thrust them suddenly back into public awareness.

From the moment the magazine issues came out, our phone never stopped ringing. Everyone called: people who knew my father personally and those who did not; people who had been arrested as part of the Doctors' Plot; those who had lain awake expecting an arrest that never came; and those who had only heard rumors. And now, this whole crowd was pressing in, trying to get into my father's party, to see him in person and to hear him speak.

In the end, we — my father, his second wife Katya, my older sister Lyalya and myself — elbowed and cajoled our way into the auditorium. The host was Eduard Beltov, who would later become an Israeli journalist by the name of Eddie Baal and who had done a brilliant job of editing my father's nearly 500-page manuscript down to the size of the excerpt for *Druzhba Narodov*.

Besides the leading lights of Soviet medicine, my father was greeted onstage by Rada Adjoubey, a daughter of Nikita Khrushchev's and editor-in-chief of the popular science magazine *Nauka i Zhizn* (*Science and Life*). Rada's magazine had published my father's first memoir essays. She became his literary "godmother."

Now, at his 90th birthday celebration, he received a wonderful surprise, perhaps the best gift he had ever received: a copy of his book *The Doctors' Plot of 1953*. The Kniga (Book) publishing house had released my father's book in its entirety on the eve of his 90th birthday, and Tamara Gromova, editor of the Kniga publishing house, formally presented it to him at the party. You should have seen how delighted he was!

My father had written that book in 1972, which was a precarious and risky time. In it, he described the history of Soviet medical professionals and intellectuals from 1917 (the year of the

Russian October Revolution) to the year he wrote the manuscript. As a prominent scientist and pathologist, he had access to inside information on certain events that were not generally known. He knew of a number of cases in which Stalin had used medicine to kill established rivals, potential rivals or people whom he simply wanted dead. He also described outrageous instances of state anti-Semitism in the Soviet Union. His work presented new evidence against the criminal Soviet regime, which made the manuscript an incredibly dangerous item to keep at home. Only our closest friends knew of its existence. We spent a long time looking for someone who could make a copy. It had to be someone who combined absolute reliability with absolute courage, since being caught undertaking such a project carried a sentence of several years' imprisonment at a labor camp. My close friend Ksana Staroselskaya, a brilliant literary translator, recommended her friend Masha Aygi. Masha came to our place and, using our Erica typewriter and carbon paper, typed the manuscript at lightning speed because she was anxious to know what came next in the story.

Masha typed up three copies (the fourth one was "blind," i.e., so faint as to be unreadable). We hid one; it became our "underground" copy, literally. We kept another copy at home for my father to make further edits and the third copy was circulated among our closest friends, who each read it quickly and passed it on — it was safer this way.

Even so, rumors began to spread around Moscow that my father had written some kind of subversive book. I dreamed of smuggling a copy out to the West. Should the book be lost, it would be a catastrophe — not only for my father personally but also for history. Of course, we could not have guessed at that time that a mere two decades later, the archives of the KGB would be opened (at least to some extent) and historians would gain access to some of the most secret information of that establishment. Since that, to us, was unimaginable, we felt that if we were to lose this manuscript to the KGB, the final, culminating moment of the Stalin era would be consigned to oblivion along with all its victims. Nevertheless, my father refused to countenance any attempts to smuggle the manuscript out to the West, believing it to be too risky for all of us. For this reason, when I made my two attempts to smuggle the copy of the manuscript out to the West, my father was not aware of them.

I tried twice and failed both times, as described below. Attempting to send such an explosive document abroad was dangerous and could easily result in years in a Soviet prison. The writers Andrey Sinyavsky and Yuli Daniel mentioned earlier had done so and paid the price, as had Aleksandr Solzhenitsyn, the man who coined the term "the Gulag Archipelago."

1. *First Attempt*

For my first attempt, a West German professor of Russian literature was my accomplice. He used to visit Moscow and brought groups of students with him. He was deeply in love with my friend Ksana Staroselskaya, and Ksana asked him for help with smuggling my father's manuscript to West Germany. The elaborate plan that we developed resembled that of a spy movie. I met my accomplice in Gorky Park and we strolled casually through the narrow alleys acting as lovers while watching for a "tail." When we were certain that we were not being followed, I gave him the manuscript, rolled up into a thick roll and wrapped in a sheet of the newspaper *Pravda*, and we parted. I was shaking in my shoes — I had just committed a terrible crime against the state, according to Soviet law. But at the same time, I also felt tremendous relief. Now, the manuscript was safe!

Unfortunately, my relief was short-lived. Several days later, my accomplice called to tell me that we must meet again at the same place in Gorky Park. He said on the phone that he had over-estimated his ability to fulfill the promise he had made to me, which I understood to mean that he wanted to give me back the manuscript. He was calling from a public phone but I knew that my phone was bugged. I was frozen with terror! This time, I put a few toiletries into my purse in case I was arrested on the spot. We met again and went through the same charade playing lovers (on shaking legs), until he returned my roll to me.

As it turned out, he had expected the West German embassy to take the manuscript from him and send it to Germany through diplomatic channels. His embassy contact refused to accept the document in hard copy but said that they might accept it if it were converted to microfilm. That, however, was utterly beyond my means. Such equipment was not accessible to private citizens and I did not know of anyone who had access to these machines at work and who might be able to help.

But at least I got away with this adventure somehow. It cost me several sleepless nights spent waiting for a knock at the door that never came. My father's manuscript remained in the Soviet Union.

2. *Second Attempt*

In the mid-1980s, at the very dawn of *perestroika*, I made my second attempt.

This story begins at the Art Museum in Budapest, where I met a wonderful American couple, Frances and Morton Clurman, with whom I would later become friends and to whom I would confide the secret of my father's manuscript.

It was my first business trip abroad. I enjoyed my time in Hungary. I fell in love with Hungarian architecture, culture, and food and spent every weekend visiting some museum in Budapest or driving out to see beautiful small towns in the vicinity.

One Saturday, I stood in front of a small painting by Marc Chagall in an otherwise empty room at the Budapest Art museum. At that time, Chagall's pictures were not exhibited in Russia, but I knew about them from reproductions in the albums that my visiting foreign colleagues used to give me. I venerated Chagall both as an exceptional artist and because my mother and great-aunt had a personal connection with the Chagall family through the city of Vitebsk. Marc Chagall was thirteen years my mother's senior.

My mother was born in a small Jewish town called Ruzhany, five hundred kilometers from Vitebsk. Her mother had died when my mom was just six, and she and her siblings had been adopted by their aunt Sophia Yakhnin who lived in Vitebsk, not far from the Chagalls. The families interacted in many ways. Aunt Sonia, a midwife, had helped a number of Marc Chagall's siblings (probably him as well) enter this world. Aunt Sonia's husband, Isaak Veincop, had a degree in pharmacology from Moscow University. His pharmacy was well known in Vitebsk and appears in one of Chagall's pictures. Chagall also later wrote in his autobiography that his father had worked in one of my Yakhnin relatives' shops where his job was to move heavy barrels of herring.

Marc Chagall became *persona non-grata* in the Soviet Union after immigrating to France. His works were not exhibited and his name was no longer mentioned. Some of his theater sketches, stored at the Bakhrushin Theater Museum in Moscow as part of the archives of the State Jewish Theater (GOSSET), were lost in a fire that occurred most likely as a result of arson.

Our family legend says that we used to own two of Chagall's sketches. They were lost along with everything else when our house was destroyed by the direct hit of a German bomb during one of the first bombing attacks on Moscow in 1941.

Let me now come back to the Budapest Art Museum where I stood alone, contemplating Chagall's painting, the only work by him that the Museum owned. I tried to imagine how the other pictures from my Chagall albums might look on the museum wall. I was so preoccupied with this mental game that I did not notice that an elderly couple had crossed the room several times before finally coming over to join me. I could see from their clothes that they were American tourists.

"What's so special about this picture that we haven't noticed? We've seen you standing here for a very long time."

Taken aback by their question, I spluttered, "But... this picture — this is a *Chagall*!"

"Yes? It's not really one of his best works..."

"I've never seen *any* other Chagall paintings in a museum."

I saw that they were amazed. Although their next question was formulated very carefully, I couldn't help but hear their puzzlement: what planet, what howling wilderness did this woman come from that she had never seen a Chagall in a museum? I explained that I was there on a business trip from Moscow. They became extremely excited. I was the first Russian they had ever met! Well, they were the first Americans I had ever met. They introduced themselves — Frances and Morton Clurman from Croton-on-Hudson, New York. Given my limited grasp of American geography, that was about as informative as telling me they were from Mars or Saturn.

Frances was a diminutive woman with bright eyes and fast movements. Morton was slightly taller than his wife and strongly built, with a sharp-eyed look that betrayed a keen sense of humor. They immediately told me that Morty had been a Trotskyite in his youth and that they were still politically aware and very concerned about, and attentive to, the situation of the Soviet Jewry. They never missed any *New York Times* articles about Soviet Jews.

Morty asked, "Why don't they exhibit Chagall in the Soviet Union? Is it because he is Jewish or because he is an emigrant?"

Later, they said that what I did next told them more about the situation in the Soviet Union than all the *New York Times* articles put together. In that room of the Budapest Art Museum, empty except for the three of us, I quickly turned my head to the left and to the right, looked around us, and only then answered, "Both."

I don't remember taking these instinctive precautions, so natural they had become for any of my Soviet contemporaries. This was early in Mikhail Gorbachev's tenure. The man he replaced, Yuri Andropov, had been a frightening throwback to our Stalinist past, and the fear that was triggered by his rule — though mercifully short-lived — was apparently still deep in my bones.

They invited me to join them for a cup of coffee and we started chatting. Morton knew plenty of American jokes; I knew lots of Russian ones. We soon realized that jokes needed no visas to travel across the ocean. Morty would start one; I would finish it. We laughed lightheartedly, pleased with each other. I was also pleased with myself; it was my first time engaging in small talk in English. They were very friendly and warm and attentive. They suggested spending the next day together. Luckily, it was a Sunday. The next day, strolling under the trees of a beautiful island in the center of Budapest, I told them my family story and the events of the Doctors' Plot. I also revealed to them the existence of my father's manuscript and my concerns about its preservation.

They excitedly promised their assistance. That night, their tourist group left by bus for Vienna. I went to see them off. Morty waved me goodbye with tears in his eyes.

Upon my return to Moscow, I found a letter from Morton telling me that their friend would be in Moscow between such and such dates and would call me from a public phone to set up a meeting. In the letter, Morty assured me that I could safely *give his friend the item* we had been talking about in Budapest because the friend was a VIP (Very Important Person) and would not be *searched at the border*. I was petrified! At that time, all incoming mail from the United States was opened and read. Morty's letter came to me in an open envelope — the KGB wanted me to know that they had already read the letter and knew I was conspiring to arrange something illegal. They could have let me go through with it and caught me red-handed but instead, for whatever reason, they opted for prevention. The day before the arrival of Morty's important friend, my home phone gave a click and stopped working. It came back to life the day after the friend's departure. Once again, the manuscript remained in Russia.

After my failed attempt to send the manuscript to America, I kept corresponding with the Clurmans using Aesopian language. I tried to explain that my telephone had suddenly *broken at the most inappropriate time* and that the problem had been so severe that it *took about a week* before I could have it repaired. I was not sure if they caught my drift.

Two years later, Morty and Frances came to visit me in Moscow. I tried to take them beyond the usual tourist spots and destinations to show them real Moscow life. They were fascinated!

Two episodes in particular from the Clurmans' visit to Moscow stick in my memory. Morty enjoyed looking into every window we passed on our walking tours. One day we passed by a grocery store located not far from my home. It was our neighborhood grocery store where my husband Volodya and I did our shopping. Morty saw a big crowd, mostly women, all crammed inside and insisted on going in. Inside, a long, snaking line of people waited to buy meat. Or rather, what passed for meat during those lean years of Socialist food shortages: dark-red, malodorous bones covered with thin layers of tendons, with some flesh peeking out here and there, lying in a heap on the counter. The women in line pushed and cursed each other, jostling for the best bones. Thinking that this was dog food, Morty asked, "Don't you have special food for dogs? American dogs wouldn't eat these bones." I explained that this meat was meant for these women and their families, and that my family also usually ate the same kind of meat. Morty couldn't believe it; it took him some time to stop weeping.

Another morning Morty came down to his hotel lobby to meet me. It was a special hotel for visiting foreigners where regular Soviet citizens like myself couldn't just walk in off the street, much less go up to a guest's room. A security guard would have asked me a million questions and kept my ID (my internal Soviet passport) until I left the hotel. Only prostitutes that paid protection money to the guards or worked for the KGB were allowed in without questioning and without surrendering their passports to the guards. So Morty came down to meet me. He looked grim. I asked what had happened. He explained that the previous night it had occurred to him to check if there was a Bible in his bedside table, like there would be in an American hotel. Opening the drawer, he found, instead of a Bible, a booklet written in English that informed him — a visiting American Jew! — that America was mired in anti-Semitism and that Jews in the United States led terrible lives, being everywhere abused and humiliated, unemployed or underpaid. "Up until last night, I never knew I lived in such atrocious conditions. I thought I lived in the best country in the world. My mistake, obviously! Perhaps I should ask for political asylum right here, in the Soviet Union," said Morty sarcastically. Soviet idiocy really knew no limits.

At the time of the Clurmans' visit to Moscow, my father's book had already been published in the Soviet Union. *Gorby* and his *Glasnost* burst upon us suddenly. It's now or never, my father decided, and in 1986, at the very beginning of *Perestroika*, I took the manuscript over to *Novy Mir* (New World), a popular magazine. The publishers of *Novy Mir* told us that they felt such a publication at that point in time would be premature. The manuscript stayed in their locked safe for about nine months. Perhaps its publication was premature today, but tomorrow it might be too late. Thus, at my father's request, I took the manuscript back from *Novy Mir* and he mailed it to *Druzhba Narodov*. A couple of days later he received a call from its editor-in-chief, Sergey Baruzdin, who was brimming with excitement:

"My dear Yakov L'vovich! Thank you so much! I've been looking all over for materials about the Doctors' Plot and was afraid that nothing had survived! This is such a gift to our magazine! We're going to get started on it right away!"

Both our publications, my father's and mine, had made quite a stir all over the world. They were immediately translated into many languages, including French, Italian, Polish, and Dutch. Dozens of documentaries were shot in our Moscow apartment by the PBS, BBC and other companies. The *New York Times* and *Washington Post* published articles that included photographs of our family. We received numerous offers from several American publishing houses. My father chose the Harvard University Press, an academic publisher. In 1991, his book, *Stalin's Last Crime: The Doctors' Plot of 1953*, prefaced with my own story, came out in the United States and England.

In 1989, as the Iron Curtain slowly lifted, I was able to return Frances and Morton's visit. The Clurmans invited me and my daughter Victoria to see them in America. It was the very first time we had ever set foot in the States. I can never adequately describe our jaw-dropping amazement after stepping out of Grand Central Station in New York and onto 42nd Street. We found ourselves in Wonderland!

During our stay with them, the Clurmans introduced me to their VIP friend who had traveled to Moscow several years ago in that failed attempt to collect my father's manuscript. His name was Leonard Shatzkin and he lived nearby in Croton-on-Hudson.

In yet another one of those implausible, believe-it-or-not coincidences, Lenny Shatzkin turned out to be a distant relative of mine! He was a nephew of my aunt Vera's (my father's sister) on her husband's side. At the time he went to Moscow, he had not known that we were related and only realized it much later, after reading personal details about my family in American newspaper reports prompted by the publication of my father's and my own revelations about the Doctors' Plot.

Lenny was a consultant for the prestigious Doubleday and McGraw Hill publishing houses. When Morty and Francis told him about meeting me in Budapest, he realized that these publishers might be interested in my father's manuscript. He flew to Moscow with a VIP status that excused him from customs searches at the airport. In Moscow, he stayed at the apartment of our mutual relative by the name of Nadya. Had he told Nadya the purpose of his visit, we could have easily met without the need for any telephone contact as my address was well known to all my relatives. But Lenny maintained a strict secrecy and did not mention my name or the purpose of his visit to anyone. Day after day, he kept trying to call me through public phones, only to hear an endless series of long beeps. Of course, he could not have known that my phone was blocked by the KGB. He finally concluded that I had gotten scared and changed my mind about sending the manuscript to America. He left Moscow feeling very disappointed and angry with me.

When we finally met at the Clurmans', I explained to Lenny what had really happened to my phone during his stay in Moscow. I had a feeling that he did not really believe me but forgave me anyway. Lenny and his wife Elkie were absolutely charming people and we struck up a life-long friendship. I eventually attended their golden wedding anniversary where he gave a memorable speech. He told a story of a young and beautiful woman who had many lovers. When parting with a regular lover, she would always ask for just one thing: a pocket knife. She never accepted any other gift. "I am very rich," said one of her lovers, "I could give you a fortune that would make you rich for the rest of your days." "No," responded the girl, "all I want is a pocket knife. Right now, I am young and beautiful and have many lovers. Yet I know that time will pass; I will lose my beauty, I will put on fat, my face will become wrinkled, and my current admirers will disappear. But I have heard that there is nothing that a boy scout won't do for a pocket knife!" With these words, Lenny presented Elkie with a small, beautifully decorated jewelry box. She opened the box and inside lay a very beautiful pocket knife with a mother-of-pearl inlaid handle!

Neither Frances and Morton Clurman nor Lenny and Elkie Shatzkin are with us anymore, but I cherish memories of them and maintain ties with their sons.

***

The stories that follow are ones I heard from my father and our friends. They are first-hand accounts of the participants of the events.

Part II

Stories From My Father
and Our Friends

4 It's Just the Plague

A person familiar with Soviet history would be justified in concluding that the main purpose of the ChK-NKVD-MGB-KGB was to arrest, torture, and kill innocent people by the millions. But there was one episode in Soviet history when the NKVD directed its efforts to saving rather than destroying people's lives. Yet, before we shed tears of sympathy, we should note that in this particular case, the NKVD operatives went into action to save their own lives along with those of others because the Black Death — yes, we are talking about the actual plague — is indifferent to ranks and shoulderboards. The laws of nature are not suspended for the NKVD.

The most incredible thing about this story is that it really happened. My father was both a witness and a participant in it. I am talking about the outbreak of the plague that occurred at the heart of Moscow during the hard freeze in December 1939. It was not the metaphorical "brown plague" as referred to by the Soviet press to the Nazis before the Molotov-Ribbentrop pact was signed. No, it was the real plague, the same Black Death that had claimed many millions of human lives throughout the centuries. Monuments for plague victims may be found in virtually any European town. The memory of the medieval epidemic still lives on in the name of one of the smaller streets at the center of Moscow: Death Alley.

Now, centuries later, the plague was once again brought to Moscow. It originated from Saratov, a provincial Russian city.

The story I am about to tell is rather mysterious. The task of investigating how the plague had come to Moscow in the middle of the 20th century was assigned to Detective Lev Sheynin. However, he was arrested very soon after receiving his assignment, at which point the investigation stopped and was never resumed.

But before I give you a detailed report of the dreadful events that threatened to ravage Moscow 75 years ago, I want to take you on a short trip into the depths of time — we will follow the trails of some of the devastating epidemics of the plague.

The earliest account of a possible plague epidemic can be found in the Bible. The Philistines of Ashdod were allegedly stricken by a plague for stealing the Arc of the Covenant in the 11th century B.C. In later centuries B.C., severe epidemics hit Ethiopia, Egypt, Libya, and Syria and eventually spread to Greece. However, any widespread disease with a high rate of mortality at that time was called a plague. Based on descriptions provided by contemporaries, some of the dreadful outbreaks could also have been caused by typhus, smallpox, or measles. The first definitive account of the plague came to be known as the "Plague of Justinian," which started in the Eastern Roman Empire in the 6th century A.D., raged for fifty years, covered a huge territory and claimed a very large number of lives. Eight centuries later, the plague returned to Europe and claimed between fifteen and twenty-five million lives. This time it reached Russia. It was during this epidemic that the first quarantine in human history was established in Venice.

The source of the plague was not known until the end of the 19th century. The first breakthrough occurred in 1894 during an epidemic in Hong Kong. Independently, two scientists, Alexandre Yersin of France and Kitasato Shibasaburo of Japan, isolated the bacteria from the bodies of plague victims and obtained their culture. Yersin noticed that human epidemics were often preceded by outbreaks of the deadly disease in rats. Finding the same bacteria in the bodies of both dead rats and human victims, he identified rats as a possible source of the bacteria. This bacterium is now called *Yersinia pestis* in honor of Yersin. The enemy had finally become visible.

Four years later, another French bacteriologist, Paul-Louis Simond, discovered that it was actually not the rats but the fleas they carried that transmitted the disease to humans. When a flea bites an infected rat, it ingests *Yersinia pestis* along with the rat's blood. Infected fleas are always hungry and bite humans to satisfy their appetite. This way, they introduce the bacteria into the human body.

The human plague takes three distinct forms: bubonic (accompanied by a characteristic swelling of the lymph nodes); pneumonic (affecting the lungs); and septicemic (a severe infection of the blood). The latter develops so fast that the victim dies before the bubonic or pneumonic forms have had time to set in.

In 1912 in Russia, doctor Ippolit Deminsky found *Yersinia pestis* in chipmunks. While culturing the bacteria, he was accidentally infected. Several hours before his death, he composed a telegram to his colleague Nikolay Klodnitsky: "Please come and take the culture. Lab notes are in order. Make autopsy of my body to confirm the transmission of disease from chipmunks to humans. Farewell. Deminsky." This was the first known case of infection with the plague in a laboratory; unfortunately, it would not be the last one.

As no drugs existed against this malady at that time, a plague diagnosis was a death sentence. Even now, despite the plethora of antibiotics available, surviving the plague is extremely rare. Just think about it: people have gone to the Moon, flights have been taken to Mars and other planets are on the horizon, but the plague has not yet been conquered despite more than a century of desperate efforts to find a solution!

About a decade ago, the city where I now live — Salt Lake City — watched with bated breath as doctors at the Primary Children's Hospital fought for the life of a 10-year-old girl who was brought to the hospital by helicopter. She lived with her family in an isolated area at the south of Utah. One summer day, her cat ran away. The girl looked for it in the desert but could not find it. After several days, the cat returned in a terrible state: it had been severely bitten and scratched, its dirty fur hung down in shreds, and a cough shook its body. The girl desperately tried to help it, but the cat died. As the girl grieved over her loss, her parents decided to send her to a scout camp in hopes that, in the company of other kids, she would forget her loss sooner. But at the camp, the girl soon became very, very sick. She developed a high fever and the same symptoms as her cat. She was taken to the hospital in Salt Lake City where the doctors made a shocking diagnosis: pneumonic plague! One could only imagine what the parents of the sick girl, as well as those of the other kids that had come in contact with her, went through. But luckily, she was the only one to get sick. Pneumonic plague is a strange infection; it becomes contagious very abruptly. Say, an hour ago, contact with a sick person was relatively safe, but an hour later, the probability of getting the disease is virtually one hundred percent.

The doctors fought for the girl's life for several months. The local newspaper and TV news ran near-daily updates on her condition. Fortunately, the girl survived; a happy ending that is almost unique in the history of the disease.

But back in the 1930s, one of the sites where the search for a cure for the plague was going on full-tilt was the city of Saratov on the banks of the Volga River in Russia. Deep in the woods, surrounded by barbed wire, stood the multi-story building of the Microbe Institute. My father suspected that the main task of the Institute was the development of a biological weapon. The plague research was highly classified, but in Russia, no secrets remain secret for too long. Saratov residents christened the Institute the "Plague Institute." One of the laboratories was dedicated to the development of an anti-plague vaccine. The head of the lab, Dr. Abram Berlin, was a brilliant and highly experienced scientist in his late thirties. He was a handsome, brave, and daring man, happily married to a very talented young pianist. His tragic death from the plague near Moscow's Red Square and the dramatic events associated with it are described below.

Dr. Berlin held a doctorate in epidemiology. After graduation, he was sent to Mongolia to organize anti-plague work there. Mongolia, an Asian country bordering Tibet, has long been considered the cradle of the plague. It is speculated that 10–15 million years ago, a Siberian marmot became the first host of *Yersinia pestis*. The Mongolians knew that tarbagans, a type of rodent similar to marmots, were responsible for the plague epidemics that occurred frequently in their country. Consequently, the Mongolians derived their own assumptions on the origins of plague epidemics that were remarkably close to the truth. During the winter, tarbagans sleep in their underground burrows. Exploiting this habit, infected weasels that carry but do not die from the plague enter the burrow and bite the host. The poison then sleeps in the tarbagan's body throughout winter. In the spring, the bitten tarbagan wakes up and gets out of his burrow. When the first thunderstorm comes and the tarbagan hears the first thunder, the poison awakens and starts acting. As the Mongolians hunt and consume tarbagans, the tarbagans transfer the poison to the hunters. After that, the disease spreads from person to person.

The Mongolians were mostly nomads. During the frequent plague epidemics, their migratory behavior spread death to themselves and others.

Dr. Berlin had to start his fight against the Mongolian plague from scratch. Three miles from the capital city, he built a small anti-plague village by the name of Tarbagan Upchin Hoto. In Mongolian, "tarbagan upchin" means "a disease caused by tarbagans." He worked non-stop, including weekends and holidays, treating and educating the Mongolian people.

Upon his return to the Soviet Union, Dr. Berlin continued his anti-plague work at the Microbe Institute in Saratov. He became the head of a lab dedicated to the development of the anti-plague vaccine. This vaccine has its own dramatic history.

Many years ago, a young girl died of the plague in Madagascar. During the post-mortem examination, plague bacteria were taken from her organs, cultured and referred to by her initials: EB. Russian scientists at the Microbe Institute obtained these bacteria and worked with them. They re-seeded them multiple times before something very curious and unexpected suddenly happened. The guinea pigs that were injected with the EB bacteria did not develop the disease. Moreover, they became immune to ordinary, highly virulent bacteria strains. The EB bacteria were alive but had lost their virulence — the EB strain had become a vaccine!

The group of scientists in Saratov decided to test this vaccine on themselves. For a long time, Moscow considered the risk to be much too high and denied permission for such an experiment. Finally, Dr. Berlin somehow persuaded the medical authorities in Moscow that it was worth trying. There were three heroes: Drs. Abram Berlin, Yevgenia Korobkova, and Victor Tumansky, the cream of the research center's crop at the Microbe Institute. After isolating themselves from the rest of the world in the basement room, their colleague Dr. Yaschshuk injected each of them with 250 million EB bacteria and left. The experiment officially started. Their colleagues and the Moscow authorities anxiously awaited the results.

The plague's incubation period is usually three to six days, but it may also be as short as 36 hours or as long as ten days. Everything went OK on the first day. On the second morning, Dr. Tumansky developed a high fever and his condition deteriorated by the hour. Was it the plague? Two stressful days passed. Finally, everyone heaved a huge sigh of relief — it turned out to be tularemia, a different disease that Dr. Tumansky had contracted many years ago. His attempted vaccination with EB had triggered a flare-up. By the third night, his fever was almost gone.

None of the participants in this unprecedented test developed the plague. After this first test, five and then eight more volunteers were injected with EB and none of them developed the disease. The results were deemed to be a complete success; the experiment ended in triumph.

From that point on, Dr. Berlin considered himself immune to the plague. He once admitted, "I have to stop working with the plague. I am too accustomed to it..."

In December 1939, the highest Soviet medical authority — the Collegium of the Commissariat for Public Health — summoned Dr. Berlin to Moscow for a report on his work. On the eve of his departure, he worked with infected guinea pigs. We will never know exactly what happened; perhaps he did not take all the necessary precautions or was too preoccupied by the upcoming trip, but he was already sick when the train from Saratov entered the Moscow railway station. He had a high fever and had started coughing. He stayed at the centrally located National Hotel on the corner of

Gorky street right next to the Red Square. He gave his report to the Collegium, but by the end of the meeting he felt really ill and was taken back to the hotel. He sent for a doctor.

The pneumonic plague generally has a sudden and well-marked onset. It initially resembles the flu or pneumonia, but a firm diagnosis cannot be given without bacteriologic examination. Still, in areas where it is endemic, it is relatively easy to identify. But who would possibly think of the plague in the middle of the 20th century at the heart of Moscow, the nation's capital? The physician who came to see Dr. Berlin was an old doctor by the name of Mikhail Russels. He had recently lost his only son, a neurosurgeon, whose plane had crashed during an expedition to the North Pole. As could be imagined, he and his wife, both in their seventies, were in deep mourning. Tired and distraught, Dr. Russels mistakenly thought that his patient had a severe form of bronchopneumonia. He sent him to the Novoyekaterininsky hospital in the center of Moscow, near Pushkin Square.

By the time of his arrival at the hospital, Dr. Berlin was already in critical condition: his face was gray, he had problems breathing, his temperature was very high, and there was blood in his sputum. That night, the doctor on duty in the emergency room was Dr. Simon Gorelik. He did not hesitate to give a diagnosis: pneumonic plague. This was a death sentence not only for Dr. Berlin but also for himself, since he had been in close contact with his patient during the stage when the disease was extremely contagious. Dr. Gorelik knew that he had no chance. He immediately isolated himself with the patient and continued treating and helping him until the patient's death. He himself died without any help, having not allowed anyone to enter his room. In his self-imposed quarantine, being already sick and knowing that he was doomed, he wrote letters to his loved ones and to Comrade Stalin. He pleaded with Stalin to release his brother who was unlawfully arrested. These letters were burned together with his body. Unfortunately, the professional and human heroism of Dr. Gorelik, a Jew, never received the recognition it deserved because of a "plague" of a different nature: Soviet anti-Semitism.

Before going into quarantine, Dr. Gorelik called the director of the Hospital to inform him that there was a plague at their facility. The director informed the Committee of State Security. The NKVD was called into action and for once was tasked with saving rather than destroying human lives. It was vitally important and urgent to identify and quarantine anyone who had come in contact with Dr. Berlin during his last 24 hours: on the train, during his presentation to the Collegium of the Commissariat for Public Health, and at the National Hotel.

To help you understand the tactics opted by the NKVD to accomplish this mission, I need to remind you that the described events were unfolding in 1939 during Stalin's purges and reign of terror. The NKVD's macabre shadow loomed over the country. Innocent people numbering in the hundreds of thousands were being taken to prisons, sent to labor camps, or shot by firing squads. Anyone might expect a late-night knock on the door, with the NKVD's raven-black car, the *voronok*, waiting outside to take the victim to the terrible Lubyanka prison in Moscow, or the "Big House" in St. Petersburg, or a local prison in a provincial city. In those years, people lost their ability to be surprised at the arrests, since no one was immune to this fate.

The plague was a different story. The government really wanted to avoid panic. Therefore, the isolation of those who had been in contact with Dr. Berlin was disguised as a series of ordinary arrests performed, as always, by the NKVD. The families of the affected individuals were not informed of the actual cause and purpose of the purported arrest; they just thought that they were losing their loved ones forever. None of them knew that these were, far more surprisingly, ten-day detentions for purposes of quarantine.

The NKVD was very efficient. As soon as it became evident what a monstrous danger had come to Moscow, emergency measures were taken to prevent the epidemic. The Novoyekaterininsky Hospital was placed on lockdown. The building was surrounded by NKVD troops, guards were posted outside all entrances and exits, no one could get out, and only persons with special permissions were allowed in. Dr. Ilya Lukomsky, the head of the oral medicine department who happened to be at the hospital at the time of Dr. Berlin's arrival, was appointed the Commandant of the clinic.

Thanks at least in part to these measures (and in part also because epidemics tend to unfold according to their own rules), the plague took only three lives: those of Drs. Berlin and Gorelik and the hospital barber who had stopped by the emergency room and approached Dr. Berlin to ask if he wanted a shave.

After these measures had been taken, a search for the people who had come in contact with Dr. Berlin began. The hospital on Sokolinaya Gora (Falcon Mountain) was cleared of patients and transformed into a quarantine facility. The entire Collegium of the Commissariat for Public Health, including its head, Dr. Georgy Mitirev, was detained and taken into quarantine. All employees of the National Hotel who might have come in contact with Dr. Berlin, as well as guests staying on the same floor, were detained. Even some of Dr. Berlin's fellow travelers from the train were found and isolated. This was the kind of thing the NKVD did well.

All this activity was performed in the strictest of secrecy to avoid panic. However, as I have already mentioned, it is very difficult to keep things secret in Russia. Rumors of the plague leaked out into the medical circles. Of course, nobody talked aloud about it. The word "plague" became taboo; those in the know never uttered it above a whisper, and even then only in a closed circle of colleagues or trusted friends to avoid being arrested for "panic-mongering." The plague in Moscow was surrounded by a conspiracy of silence.

Meanwhile, the detentions could not remain hidden from the public for long. Rumors of the arrests of the Commissariat for Public Health's top leadership, including its Head, began spreading around Moscow like wildfire. On one level, this was nothing new; Stalin had long made a practice of arresting groups of people connected by a common profession, claiming to discover one conspiracy after another among archeologists, philosophers, and highest-ranking army commanders, just to name a few. The public became accustomed to these trials. But the arrests of top-level public health officials, though not publicly announced, were certainly extremely frightening, sparking rumors that drugs in pharmacies were poisoned and doctors were not to be trusted. This was a dress rehearsal for the terrible events surrounding the Doctors' Plot of 1952–1953 — the last of Stalin's crimes that would shock the country fourteen years later.

Since the news of the plague was no longer a secret in medical circles, my father was not surprised when he got a call in the middle of the night from the Deputy People's Commissar for Public Health, Sergey Kolesnikov, who had replaced the isolated Commissar Mitirev. Kolesnikov asked my father to report immediately to the Health Department. He said that he could not explain over the phone why my father was so urgently needed, but my parents guessed the reason correctly anyway. A car was sent for my father and he arrived at the Health Department at about 1 a.m. The situation there was reminiscent of wartime. Kolesnikov briefed my father on the main events and asked him to perform an autopsy on the patient who had died in the Novoyekaterininsky hospital, allegedly of pneumonic plague. My father agreed to perform the autopsy on condition that he would not be placed in quarantine. His condition was accepted.

Dad was struck by what he saw on his arrival at the Novoyekaterininsky hospital. Soldiers, armed with rifles and dressed in floor-length sheepskin coats, guarded the gate and the entrance to the building. Other soldiers were warming themselves around small fires in the hospital yard. Inside the hospital there was an ominous silence.

The Commandant of the hospital, Dr. Lukomsky, was an old friend of my father's. He met him at the door and took him to his office. They drank tea and chatted while waiting for the bacteriologist who had to be on hand to take the autopsy materials for evaluation.

The autopsy was performed in a very unusual manner: the body had been put into a resin-impregnated coffin located in a special isolation ward. These circumstances were quite disturbing, even to a professional. After the autopsy was over, my father took all the necessary precautions for decontamination and started walking back to the room where he had left his clothes. He had hardly crossed the threshold when he heard a click and realized that he had been locked in. Exhausted after a sleepless and stressful night, he started pounding on the door demanding to be let out immediately. The voice on the other side answered that he had no authority to let him out. My father then asked them for just two things: to have a cup of tea and to get in touch with the Department of Public Health to confirm their agreement that he would not be kept under quarantine. Both requests were satisfied. First, the lock clicked again and a cup of tea was pushed in through a tiny crack in the door. A little while later, Dr. Lukomsky entered the room and informed my father that he was free to go.

He drove to his lab to take another good shower and then called my mother asking for fresh underwear and a different suit. After that, they finally went back to the cramped space we called home.

Anxious and exhausted, my father came home, but he had barely gone back to sleep when he was awakened by another telephone call. My mother answered the call. The voice on the other end told her that the mayor of Moscow had already sent a car to take my father to the First City Hospital to perform a very important autopsy. My mother responded with a categorical refusal, explaining that my father was sleeping after a very difficult night. Still, half an hour later, there was a knock on the door, followed by a heated argument between my mother and the newcomers. They told her that a patient had died of the plague in a surgical clinic at the First City Hospital and the clinic was already under quarantine. My father was needed to perform an autopsy and confirm the diagnosis of the plague. My mother objected: "Are there no other experienced pathologists in Moscow?" to which one of the callers responded as follows: "We cannot let all our pathologists get infected with the plague now can we?" My mother was a very polite, kind and peaceful person but the callousness of this response infuriated her. Meanwhile, my father decided that he had to take this new assignment. He was a consultant at the First City Hospital and the hospital was clearly in trouble. He had no doubt that there was no plague at this clinic and it was all just nonsense triggered by the panic.

The First City Hospital was surrounded by armed soldiers. A very grim, depressing atmosphere reigned inside the surgical clinic. There was dead silence. The nurses wore double gowns with many-layered, full masks hiding their faces; they wandered along the empty corridors like shadows.

A duty doctor told my father what happened. The day before, a young man had been operated on at the clinic to remove a stomach ulcer. The next morning, the patient's condition worsened: he developed a high fever and severe peritoneal pain. A consultant was called in to the clinic. He lifted the sheet, saw the rash covering the patient's body, dropped the sheet, cried: "It's the plague!" and ran away. The dreaded word had been uttered and the wheel of mortal fear was set in motion. Nobody dared to approach the patient. He remained without any help and soon died.

(As an aside, the consultant, that poor excuse for a doctor, was later promoted to the position of Chief Oncologist of the USSR. One famous physician commented on his appointment by saying: "We wrote advanced courses for oncology students but forgot to mention that the Chief Oncologist is allowed to know nothing!")

My father suspected from the very beginning that what was going on there was behavior characteristic of inexperienced and unthinking surgeons. When something goes wrong after the surgery, they reach for any other explanation — the flu, or meningitis — except post-surgical complications caused by the surgeon's incompetence. He was right. The autopsy confirmed his suspicions: the patient had died of peritonitis accompanied by general sepsis and hemorrhagic rash.

After the autopsy, normal life at the clinic was quickly restored. The nurses took off their masks and became pretty and cheerful. The hospital gates reopened to admit patients who needed urgent care but had been deprived of it. This is what fear, panic, and one single moron can do to a large human population!

There were a few more false alarms, but fortunately no more plague cases.

While recounting this story to us, my father concluded with a recollection of his conversation with Dr. Lukomsky at the Novoyekaterininsky hospital where, as the reader may remember, they drank tea before conducting the autopsy on Dr. Berlin. The protagonist of this episode was the old Dr. Russels who, after sending Dr. Berlin to the hospital with the erroneous diagnosis of bronchopneumonia, had forgotten all about him. As he grieved the loss of his son, the patient completely slipped his mind. Therefore, he was stunned to hear the pounding on his door the next night. The knock on the door in the middle of the night could mean only one thing: the NKVD was coming to arrest him; there was not much room for other interpretations. Dr. Russels opened the door and received confirmation of his fears in the form of two NKVD visitors, who ordered him to follow them.

What was the poor man to think? He tried to comfort his wife by insisting that this must be a mistake, that he was not guilty of anything, that this misunderstanding would soon be cleared up. But, then, hadn't hundreds of thousands of people before him uttered these same words in a similar situation? His wife started packing his things: warm clothes, a toothbrush etc. — all the prison essentials that the Russians of that time, with their perennial black humor, had dubbed "a gentleman's carry." The visitors told her that he would not need anything, but Dr. Russels insisted on taking the package with him: "I know what people need *over there*."

On his way, accompanied by the two NKVD men, he searched his memory desperately as he tried to figure out what could have led to his arrest. He could not find anything. He even started wondering whether his arrest might be somehow related to the tragic death of his son. Was he being posthumously implicated in some sort of wrongdoing?

His contemplations were interrupted by their arrival at the Novoyekaterininsky hospital. It was only there that poor Dr. Russels was informed by Dr. Lukomsky of the exact reason for his "arrest" and the nature of the disease his unfortunate patient had carried. Dr. Russels realized at last that this was not a real arrest. Excited beyond words, he pleaded with Dr. Lukomsky to allow him to make a call to his wife, whom he had left in complete despair. Dr. Lukomsky allowed him to make the call. With trembling hands, Dr. Russels dialed the number and in an exultant, triumphant voice shouted these exact words into the telephone:

"My dear, it's me! I'm calling from the Novoyekaterininsky hospital. They suspect that I may have caught the plague from a patient of mine. So don't worry! It's not this horrible thing we thought it was! *It's just the plague!*"

****

After the events described above, the expression "isolation into quarantine" entered the Russian vernacular as a euphemism for the dangerous word "arrest." In Stalin's era, both conveyed the concept of disaster that might strike anyone at any time, leaving them powerless to resist. In Russia, the word "freedom" was never part of the vocabulary, and until today still isn't. Sadly, the Stalinist "plague" is still virulent in Russia, producing periodic ugly and frightening outbreaks.

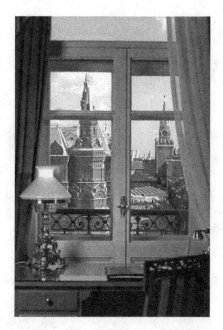

A view from the window of the National Hotel where the plague patient Dr. Berlin stayed.

5

Chapter

Academician Vassily Parin and the Anti-Cancer Vaccine *KR*

At the end of the 1940s, the medical world in Moscow was shaken by sensational news. Two well-known and respected microbiologists, Nina Klyuyeva and Grigory Roskin, announced that they had developed a preparation that was capable of curing various types of cancer. They called it KR (this preparation was later known in pharmacology as *"Cruzin"* or CR after its source, *Trypanosoma cruzi*).

Trypanosoma cruzi is a parasite that lives in the gastro-intestinal tract of the "kissing bug." The insect is so called because it prefers to bite humans on the lips, specifically at the border between the skin and mucous membranes. The bite introduces the parasite into the human body where it is carried by the bloodstream to various organs, destroying host cells.

This fact was the logical starting point for Klyuyeva and Roskin's theory. Starting in the mid-1920s, Klyuyeva and Roskin were running their experiments on mice with inoculated breast cancer. The scientists found that when the *Trypanosoma cruzi* parasites were injected into the bloodstream of cancerous mice, they were selectively accumulated in the tumors, killing cancerous cells. Importantly, this tumor-destroying ability was retained by dead parasites.

The results of their experiments in mice were so encouraging that Klyuyeva and Roskin organized human trials spanning a wide variety of cancer types. Their clinical trial results did not allow rigorous statistical analysis; yet, the researchers considered them positive. In 1946, Klyuyeva and Roskin described their work in a monograph entitled *The Biotherapy of Cancer*, which was published in the USSR.

The authors wanted to publish their manuscript in the West. They were aware that the founder and the first Academician Secretary of the Academy of Medical Sciences of the USSR, Dr. Vassily Vassilievich Parin, was about to fly to the United States for a scientific exchange and that his mission had been approved by Stalin himself.

The Soviet Union had just received a gift of an entire industrial production line of penicillin from America, its erstwhile ally in the recent war. Seeking an appropriate return gesture, the People's Commissar for Health approved Klyuyeva and Roskin's request and instructed Dr. Parin to present about the *KR* vaccine to the Americans, give them a sample, and offer Klyuyeva and Roskin's monograph for publication in the United States. Hence, Klyuyeva and Roskin handed their manuscript to Dr. Parin.

In the Soviet Union, excitement about the *KR* vaccine spilled over more broadly beyond medical circles. The Soviet government became interested in the anti-cancer vaccine, considering it a trump card in their political game. Stalin read the manuscript and wrote in the margins: "Invaluable work!" That was when it was discovered that Klyuyeva and Roskin had handed their manuscript to Dr. Parin, who had offered it to American publishers.

Upon Dr. Parin's return, both he and the creators of the vaccine were summoned to the Kremlin to explain themselves.

The meeting was considered so important that Stalin himself was present from the beginning to the end.

The exceptional value of the discovery was not in doubt. The meeting was called to discuss how this work had found its way to the U.S. before the leaders of the Soviet Party and State had a chance to familiarize themselves with it. The authors were accused of cosmopolitanism, vanity, and slavish adulation of the West. Suddenly, Stalin turned to Dr. Roskin and asked:

"Do you trust Parin?"

"I do," answered Roskin.

Stalin addressed the same question to Dr. Klyuyeva.

"I do," answered Klyuyeva.

"And I don't," concluded Stalin, and Dr. Parin's fate was sealed. In 1947, he was arrested and sentenced to twenty-five years in prison. His three-month trip to America "for continuation of mutual exchange of scientific information" landed him in the horrible Vladimirskaya prison.

In contrast, Klyuyeva and Roskin were not arrested in order not to jeopardize their valuable research. They were let off with a "court of honor," a public proceeding designed to shame them before their peers and the general public.

The "court of honor" took place at the Moscow Variety Theater and attracted a crowd larger than the Theater's best shows ever did. It was prefaced with an appropriately theatrical introduction that detailed how an evil traitor and spy had seduced two strayed lambs. The lambs, of course, were Klyuyeva and Roskin, and the traitor and spy was Dr. Parin.

Klyuyeva and Roskin asked my father to serve as an expert for their clinical trials. Unfortunately, as is not uncommon, the *KR* vaccine, although very active in a test tube and in mice, proved useless against tumors in the human body. This was the conclusion my father came to.

Klyuyeva and Roskin were trapped. Indeed, who would dare declare KR ineffective after Stalin himself had called it invaluable! A public admission of this fact was tantamount to suicide. Only my recklessly brave father dared… and miraculously got away with it. He was summoned to the Kremlin and ordered to present his reasons for concluding that KR was ineffective on humans. He gave such a clear explanation that even the Politburo members understood it and let him go (albeit not for long). My father's conclusions were later confirmed by other government experts in large-scale clinical trials, and work on *KR* stopped. The great anti-cancer vaccine, regrettably, became the discovery that never was… I need to add that Klyuyeva and Roskin's manuscript was never published in the USA due to the low quality of their initial clinical trials. Grigory Roskin soon died of a heart attack; Nina Klyuyeva outlived him by seven years.

Klyuyeva and Roskin, the scientists with a tragic story, inspired the founding of cancer biotherapy, a promising field in current biomedical research. Their idea has lived on.

Academician Parin spent seven years in Vladimirskaya prison where he was subjected to horrible humiliation and tortures. His keepers beat him, used threats against his children to blackmail him, and kept him in a solitary confinement cell for some time.

Dr. Parin was one of the first to return from the Gulag after Stalin's death. In 1955, he was fully rehabilitated and re-elected as Academician Secretary of the Medical Academy. More will be told about his after-prison years in Chapter 7, "Mischka."

The Death of Andrey Sakharov

At his 90th birthday celebration, my father said, "I'm beginning to suspect that I may be getting old." He was not being coy. In his 90s, he neither looked nor acted old. He remained physically and professionally active almost to the very end of his remarkable life.

His last professional appearance came at the age of 91. Fifty years, almost to the day, after my father had performed the plague-related autopsies, he was asked to participate in Andrey Sakharov's autopsy — another assignment of great social importance.

Although some readers may be unfamiliar with it, in the second half of the 20th century, the name Andrey Sakharov was known all over the world. According to the Center for the History of Physics (CHP), a division of the American Institute of Physics:

Andrey Dmitrievich Sakharov (1921–1989) was a Soviet physicist who became, in the words of the Nobel Peace Committee, a spokesman for the conscience of mankind. He was fascinated by fundamental physics and cosmology, but first he spent two decades designing nuclear weapons. He came to be regarded as the father of the Soviet hydrogen bomb, contributing perhaps more than anyone else to the military might of the USSR. But gradually Sakharov became one of the regime's most courageous critics, a defender of human rights and democracy. He could not be silenced, and helped bring down one of history's most powerful dictatorships.[1]

A leading designer of the Soviet H-bomb, Sakharov underwent a crisis of conscience after he realized the deadly consequences of his work. In 1968, his essay entitled "Reflections on Progress, Peaceful Coexistence, and Intellectual Freedom," an attack on the Soviet political system, was published in the West. In 1975, Sakharov was awarded the Nobel Peace Prize. In 1980, he denounced the Soviet military intervention in Afghanistan and was banished to internal exile in the town of Gorky to silence his opposition to the regime. His exile was lifted in December 1986 by Mikhail Gorbachev, then head of the Soviet Union and the author of the new Soviet policy of reform and openness (*perestroika* and *glasnost*). Gorbachev allowed Sakharov to return to Moscow.

Sakharov continued to promote democracy in the Soviet Union for the rest of his life. He was elected to the Soviet Congress (the Congress of the People's Deputies) and was active in the Soviet human-rights society, *The Memorial*, that he co-founded in January 1989 and chaired until his death. He died on December 14, 1989, after giving a speech before the Soviet Congress calling for political pluralism, a market economy, and opposition against the Soviet war in Afghanistan.

In the early morning of December 15, 1989, I was awakened by a telephone call from my friend Irina, wife of Yuli Daniel. Through her sobbing, I could barely recognize two words: "Andrei Dmitrievich." Sakharov — dead? This was a terrible loss. It is hard to convey Andrei Sakharov's central role and importance to the Soviet people of my generation, especially that of my circle of friends. At that time, at the dawn of *perestroika*, his name had

---

[1] https://history.aip.org/history/exhibits/sakharov/

come to symbolize our collective hope that the Soviet Union could be redeemed and transformed into a "normal" country with freedom, fairness and dignity for all.

To me and my friends, he meant all that and more — not just a name on our banner but an exhausted man I used to greet, with his wife Yelena Bonner, at *Memorial* meetings. For us, his death was a personal tragedy that seemed especially ominous because just earlier that day, millions of Soviet TV viewers watching the proceedings of the Soviet Congress witnessed Mikhail Gorbachev being appallingly rude to him, even shutting off Sakharov's microphone to cut short his controversial speech. Although Gorbachev had brought Sakharov back from his exile in Gorky, their relationship remained strained. On that day, Sakharov said that he would, shortly, publicly declare his formal political opposition to Gorbachev.

Now this would never happen because he was dead.

Several days later, when Yelena Bonner came to our home to ask my father about the results of the autopsy, she described to my father and me the circumstances of Sakharov's death — very odd, if not downright suspicious. The family lived in a two-room apartment in a tall building and used another identical apartment located one floor below as Sakharov's study. After dinner, he told Yelena that he was going to take a nap before working on his speech for the next day. He asked her to wake him up in an hour and a half and went downstairs to his study. When she went downstairs an hour and a half later, the door of the apartment was wide open and he was lying across the doorstep, dead.

Yelena Bonner's cries were answered by two young men who had been standing out on a landing, smoking. They lifted Sakharov, put him on the couch and tried, futilely, to perform CPR on him even though there was no doubt that he was already dead. They then called for an ambulance, which arrived two and a half *hours* later. The doctors officially pronounced Sakharov dead, but it was clear that he had died instantly, perhaps less than a minute after he had parted with his wife on the porch of their apartment.

Because Sakharov had been a member of the Soviet Academy of Sciences and a prominent political figure, his death was announced on the official radio newscast. My father wrote in his notes: "At the tragic moment when I heard about Sakharov's death, the words of the Easter Liturgy sprang to mind: *Trampling down death by death.* Sakharov's words were already barely audible amid the noise of our clamoring world. They were drowned out by an onslaught of vulgar political crudeness."

Given the politically significant timing of his death and the fact that the family never locked their doors, people were bound to wonder if he had been murdered. An autopsy was deemed necessary to rule out foul play.

Several hours after the official announcement of Sakharov's death, Yuri Vassiliev, a family friend of the Sakharovs, phoned my father. Forty years prior, Vassiliev had been a Ph.D. student at the Institute of Morphology where my father served as deputy-director. In the intervening years, Vassiliev had become a well-known scientist. He said that he was calling at the request of both Yelena Bonner and Sakharov's Academy colleagues, who wanted my father to attend the autopsy in the hope that his presence — as a leading pathologist of his time as well as a man known for his integrity — would prevent any attempt to hide the cause of death should it turn out to be a homicide.

The day after the autopsy, my father began writing down his notes. I present them at the end of this chapter, slightly edited to simplify the scientific terminology.

At my father's request, I accompanied him to the Kremlin morgue where Sakharov's body awaited us. Once denied access to the Kremlin hospital as a patient, the great man had finally entered it as a corpse.

We drove through a horrible snowstorm. When we finally pulled up, we saw several police cars circling the building, their blue and red lights searching silently through a wall of snow. Even in death, Sakharov was perceived as a threat.

When we made it to the entrance, uniformed guards did not want to let me in. I said that I would only leave if my father accompanied me, and if I did, the next day it would be all over the media everywhere that the pathologist brought in for the autopsy by Sakharov's widow had been denied access to the building. This argument convinced them: the last thing they wanted was speculation about the cause of Andrey Sakharov's death, so they let me in.

1. *Andrei Sakharov's autopsy: A View From the Hallway of the Kremlin Morgue*

An officer took me to the office of Professor Postnov, the Head of the Pathology Department of the Kremlin hospital. I was ordered to stay there and not leave the room. Other officers took my father somewhere.

I was liberated by Professor Postnov himself. About an hour after the autopsy had begun, he opened his door and was startled to find me there.

> "What are you doing here?"
> "An officer in uniform brought me in here and told me to stay put."
> "They're not in charge here — *I'm* in charge here! You should feel free to go anywhere you like. If you like, you can be in the operating hall near your father."

"Oh no, thank you, I'd rather not. But if I may ask, what have you found?"

"Nothing yet. Based on the circumstances of the death, we were expecting a massive heart attack, but it doesn't look like that was the case. We haven't opened the heart yet, but based on what we've seen so far, I don't think he had a heart attack. More likely he had a stroke."

Postnov picked up the phone. I stepped out so as not to eavesdrop, but the building was so silent that I could not help but overhear him. He repeated the information he had just given me. I had missed the beginning of his call and could not tell whom he was calling but, based on his tone, I believe it was Mikhail Gorbachev himself.

During the course of the autopsy, Postnov made several similar calls, relaying the findings as they unfolded. The authorities were understandably anxious to know whether this was a death from natural causes. The alternative — a murder — would have been very damaging to Gorbachev's reputation and advantageous for his enemies. On the eve of Sakharov's expected announcement of his formal opposition to Gorbachev, after the ugly scene at the Soviet Congress that had been seen by millions on TV, many would have been prepared to believe that Gorbachev himself had ordered Sakharov's murder.

After Postnov had released me, I wandered along the hallway. The participants of the autopsy took turns stepping out of the operating hall. They gave me their news and information about my father. The autopsy took a very long time, about six hours; my 91-year-old father spent all that time standing at the autopsy table.

Several hours had passed since the start of the autopsy, but the cause of death still remained unclear. With each passing hour, the pathologists looked ever more anxious. There was a brief but intense moment of panic. A young man in uniform rushed out of the operating hall and sprinted down the hallway. When he reached me, he exclaimed, "We've found something unprecedented!" — and ran on. Luckily, the panic was short-lived. Later, on our way back, my father explained to me that the panic had been caused by the discovery of blood clots inside the bones of Sakharov's skull and on the surface of his brain. Had he been killed by a blow to the head? My father, who was the first to recover, noticed that the blood they were seeing was actually very old, but the moment was really dramatic...

In the end, the autopsy did not reveal any of the typical causes of sudden death: no heart attack, no rupture of the aorta, no embolism of a pulmonary artery, and no stroke. Even more surprisingly, there were no traces of earlier strokes either, though after his return from exile in Gorky, Sakharov certainly looked like a person who had suffered a stroke. Yelena Bonner explained to us later that the stroke-like symptoms appeared after Sakharov had been forcibly hospitalized in Gorky. The authorities hospitalized him to put an end to the hunger strike he had undertaken to protest their refusal to allow Yelena to seek medical treatment in the USA. Upon his discharge from the hospital, his gait had altered and become unsteady, his handwriting had also changed, and his jaw had begun to tremble uncontrollably. These symptoms, called extrapyramidal syndromes, certainly resembled those of a stroke, but they were also similar to those that can be induced by overdoses of some psychotropic drugs, such as the phenothiazine-thioxantene group of agents. Was Sakharov forcibly administered these drugs during his stay at the Gorky hospital? Since the Soviet regime was known to do this to political opponents and dissidents (this kind of forcible hospitalization and medication had become known as "punitive psychiatry"), this assumption appears quite likely.

After the autopsy, the participants gathered in a small room to discuss the results. I heard the whole discussion. The doctors were apparently stymied. What should they put down as the cause of death? Due to the absence of evidence, the possibility of violent death was not discussed.

Sakharov's physician from the hospital of the Academy of Sciences insisted that he had suffered from an ischemic disease and died from a heart attack. The pathologists objected: neither ischemic disease nor a heart attack had been confirmed by the autopsy. Or, to be precise, he did have heart disease, but he did not die from a heart attack.

The discussion lasted a long time until my father said:

"I have almost no doubts that Andrey Dmitrievich suffered from cardiomyopathy. Cardiomyopathy can cause sudden death resulting from an irregular heartbeat. We did not find any convincing proof of violent death, so I think that Andrey Dmitrievich had died from cardiac arrest caused by cardiomyopathy. However, only a histological examination of the heart may confirm or disprove this diagnosis."

With great relief, the majority agreed with this conclusion.

By the time we were driven back home, it was late at night. In the car, my father kept discussing the results of the autopsy. He was surprised by the relatively good condition of Sakharov's cardiovascular system. He said with sadness: "If Andrey Dmitrievich had not died yesterday, he could have lived many more years... though of course a heart as sick as that could also have stopped at any moment. A slight push on the chest, by accident, would probably have been enough to stop his heart. He had a 'tired' heart."

My friends later asked me whether, given his advanced age, my father might have missed something during the autopsy. I answered without any reservation: no, he could not have. He was a consummate professional. His professional eye had remained sharp and his memory undimmed almost to the day of his death at the age of ninety-seven and a half, which never ceases to amaze me and everyone else who knew him. On top of that, his rigorous, old-school notions of civic honor and responsibility made him approach the autopsy with utmost care and attention.

2. *Excerpts from Yakov Rapoport's Notes*

This assignment was tremendously challenging — emotionally, physically, and ethically. It was going to be a test of my professional skill. In the course of the autopsy many sensitive moments could arise that would require quick solutions. I was 91, and my physical condition was far from ideal: my range of movement limited, my endurance not what it once was. But I did not hesitate for more than a few seconds. I said yes.

Shortly after Vassiliev's call, I received a call from a colleague of Sakharov's, Dr. Fradkin, a physicist. He asked permission to visit me in order to discuss the details of my assignment. He came by at about 3 pm. He explained why they had chosen me and what they expected of me. What he told me further reinforced my decision to participate; it was as though this work had been entrusted to me by Andrey Dmitrievich himself, who was reaching out to me to help solve the mystery of his death… I accepted this task as the highest honor of my life.

Fradkin told me the details. Contrary to my expectations, the autopsy was going to be performed at the pathology department of the Kremlin Hospital in Kuntzevo rather than the small pathology department at the Hospital of the Academy of Sciences, where autopsies of Academy employees were normally performed and where I had paid my last respect to my late friend, physicist Lev Landau.

Another surprise was that besides the dissector and myself, the autopsy would be attended by three other pathologists, members of the Medical Academy. I became concerned: wouldn't it cause a clash of ambitions? I asked Dr. Fradkin if the others were aware that I had been invited. He assured me that they were not only aware but they were actually very glad that I was going to participate. Even the prosecutor was in agreement, expecting that my presence would lay to rest any conspiracy theories on the cause of Andrey Sakharov's death.

I asked my younger daughter, Natasha, to accompany me. She agreed, as I had expected. At about 4 pm two young men (one of them a veritable giant) arrived to pick us up, and off we went — in deep darkness, through an epic snowstorm, looking for the Kremlin morgue. Our driver did not know the way. I became concerned that we would be late, but my companions reassured me that the people in charge had agreed that the autopsy would not begin without me. It was about 6 pm by the time we finally arrived. There, a new surprise awaited: the morgue looked dramatically different from the modest facility at the Academy of Sciences. The Kremlin morgue was a grand, brand new, beautiful building.

We made our way through a large, empty autopsy room. Only one table was occupied. Several people were scurrying around at the head of the corpse laid out on the table. I asked what they were doing and was told that they were taking a cast from Sakharov's face and hand for the death mask. Judging by the position of his head, they were close to being finished. I was shocked, because the preparations and manipulations involved in the making of a death mask could significantly affect or obscure vital details of the autopsy. From this, I concluded that they were proceeding on the assumption that Sakharov's death had been brought about by natural causes. Knowing what I did about the circumstances of his death, this assumption surprised me.

My companions led me down a wide hallway which had many doors opening into it. We arrived at a large office with a big desk abutting a long conference table. There I saw and recognized my three colleagues. They were: Yu. R. Postnov, Head of Pathology at the Kremlin Hospital; V. V. Serov, Chair of the Pathology department at the 1st Medical Institute; and I. K. Permyakov, Head of Pathology at the Sklifosovsky Institute of Emergency Medicine. They greeted me very warmly. There was no sign of the competing ambitions I had been concerned about. They were drinking tea, and Serov poured me a cup and offered imported biscuits and chocolate.[2] Also present were two nondescript staffers who, judging by their uniform, were with the public prosecutor's office. One of them was apparently the prosecutor who had approved my participation in the autopsy. Besides them, there was a heavy-set lieutenant-general with Army shoulderboards. He looked unfriendly and hostile and was clearly not happy with my arrival. I asked who he was and was told he was "Tomilin," as though I was expected to know this name, but it did not ring any bells. My colleagues explained that he was head of forensic medicine at both the 1st Medical Institute and the Academy of the Ministry of Internal Affairs.

My colleagues told me that the autopsy would be performed by forensic personnel. From this I understood that my colleagues and I were there to attend as consultants but not to take part in the actual autopsy. I knew that my job was to make sure that, if Sakharov's death was in fact the result of a criminal act, the people performing the autopsy did not attempt to conceal that fact. I wondered whether my colleagues had been brought in for the opposite purpose. I did hope that they were not biased, although hoping for

---

[2] These were a rare treat at that time of food shortages. — NR

professional integrity in the context of our Soviet history since the October Revolution might be the height of naïveté.

After the death cast was taken, we were invited into the autopsy hall. The autopsy was performed by the forensic expert, who was a tall man of about forty. I don't know his name, but he was clearly an expert in both performing the autopsy and describing the anatomical findings. He listened to us and responded to our requests without any objections. He demonstrated to us the details of the organs and their changes and often asked us to confirm his conclusions. All in all, he appeared to me to be an experienced dissector who dictated his findings in good faith without trying to hide any details that could have been significant for the final diagnosis. He was in charge there while we — the pathologists and even the two-star general — were present as mere consultants, each in his specialized field.

During the autopsy, a woman photographer took many photographs; she appeared to be very experienced in forensic medicine.

Pathologists deal with cases of sudden death fairly often; in these cases, their field intersects with that of forensic medicine (except for cases where the cause of death is not in doubt). In the first decade of the 20th century, Professor Pyotr Minakov was the king of Russian forensic medicine. His fascinating lectures were attended by thousands of listeners, many of whom had no connection to the medical field but were attracted by both the depth and breadth of his discussions of forensic problems. He founded the Russian school of forensic medics. In recent decades, forensic medicine has taken a giant step forward. Revolutionary advances in technology have provided it with a vast repertoire of methods, such that I would venture to claim that violent death can no longer escape the eye of a forensic expert.

I will omit a detailed description of our examination of Sakharov's organs and systems and highlight only the most salient findings. These findings concerned, primarily, the condition of the cardio-vascular and central nervous systems, the respiratory system and certain other systems that perform an overall regulatory function in the body.

The first phase of the autopsy failed to reveal the degree of damage to the vital organs we had anticipated. There was, for instance, no pronounced sclerosis of major arteries, no rupture of the arteries, no fatal internal bleeding or aspiration, etc. None of the usual causes of instantaneous death were apparent. The lungs were filled with air, the blood supply to the lungs appeared sufficient, and the airways did not contain any vomited mass. Remarkably, neither the aorta nor its major branches showed the kind of changes that might be expected and observed in a man of nearly seventy years of age.

The relative morphological integrity of the major arteries of Sakharov's coronary system was unexpected because it was inconsistent with his medical records on file with the hospital of the Academy of Sciences, which documented Sakharov as suffering from recurrent angina pectoris of ischemic origin. However, Sakharov's wife, Yelena Bonner, an experienced doctor who had observed his attacks of chest pain for many years, told me later in a personal meeting that his chest pains were inconsistent with those normally associated with angina pectoris. His pain did not radiate to the left shoulder or arm and was easily treated with simple drugs like Validol.

Similarly, while we had expected to find the kind of pathology typical of chronic coronary heart disease, our expectations were not confirmed. To be honest, the appearance of the heart when examined with the naked eye was also something of a puzzle. We had expected to find more distinct and clear morphological evidence of sudden death. The heart, once removed, was found to be uniformly enlarged, weighing 560.0 g — almost double the weight of an average heart. Despite the visible hypertrophy of the heart, the cardiac muscle was uniformly flaccid. Upon dissection, the cavities of the heart were found to contain a small number of small blood clots.

Before the skull was opened, I suggested to the two-star general that Sakharov's brain should not be dissected after extraction but should be transferred, intact, to the Brain Institute for purposes of study. As the deceased had been a person of extraordinary intellectual and psychological qualities, I believed that his brain should be examined by specialists. I told the general about my autopsy of Lev Landau, whose brain I had extracted, preserved in formalin and given to the Brain Institute for dissection, which had been conducted also in my presence. Of course, Landau's autopsy was not forensic in nature.

The two-star general considered my suggestion with visible reservations but eventually passed it on to the medical expert performing the autopsy. However, as soon as the skull was removed and the surfaces of the skull and the brain were exposed, it became apparent that my suggestion could not be carried out. What we saw was striking, even shocking. This was the first time in my nearly seventy years of practice that I witnessed anything like this. Multiple blood-red spots, varying in size between 1 and 4 cm, were scattered around within the dense bone of the removed cranial cover; they looked as if they were embedded in the bone. No one counted them. They were irregularly shaped and looked like fuzzy stains; some of them were of a pinkish color, others distinctly red. I suggested taking an X-ray of the bone but that turned out to be impossible because the pathology department did not have the necessary equipment. It was around 11 pm and X-ray facilities at other departments were closed.

Various hypotheses on the origin of these inclusions into the dense and compact bone tissue were put forth and almost instantly rejected. The suggestion that these were Paccioni's granulations[3] appeared most plausible, and its proponent took a fragment of the cut bone for an eventual histological examination of the most expressive spot.

The surface of the cerebral hemispheres, especially that of the left hemisphere, also presented an unusual appearance. It was covered with a dense membrane, 2 to 3 mm in thickness, formed by a fibrous tissue with a brownish hue.

Although Sakharov's brain was dissected in the ordinary manner which caused a severe loss of integrity, it was nevertheless transferred to the Brain Institute.

In the days that followed, I could not stop thinking about the mysterious incrustations in the bones of Sakharov's skull and on the surface of the left hemisphere. There was one other anomaly: a transverse scar that crossed the frontal bone. I thought that these findings were most consistent with a birth trauma. Yelena Georgiyevna came to visit me a week after Andrey Dmitrievich's death and I asked her whether he had experienced any kind of trauma at birth. She answered without hesitation that, based on the recollections of a close relative who had known Andrey Dmitrievich since birth, he had indeed suffered a severe birth trauma. In a letter written on May 23, 1921, two days after Sakharov's birth, his

---

[3] Granulation tissue is a connective tissue enriched with blood vessels and young cells; it is formed in the process of wound healing.

uncle had written to his godmother that "the delivery was of second degree in terms of complexity." Sakharov entered this world after a very difficult delivery that resulted in a cephalohematoma (hematoma of the skull). Yelena Georgiyevna told me that in his baby pictures, up until the age of one or so, Sakharov always wore a headscarf that hid his cranial deformity.

However, I paid so much attention to the changes in Sakharov's skull and brain simply because they belonged to an extraordinary person. They played no role in his sudden death and are not relevant to it.

What, then, was the cause of his sudden death? Though his heart did not present clear morphological evidence of sudden death, its appearance was indicative of cardiomyopathy, which had been recognized as a distinct disease as recently as the 1970s. Since that time, cardiomyopathy has been extensively discussed in medical literature throughout the world. In 1976, cardiomyopathy entered Soviet medical literature through the publication of my own research in the field.

Cardiomyopathy may be the result of various pathogenic factors. Sakharov experienced a wide variety of them in his life, including severe neuro-psychological stress. Infections and allergies should not be disregarded either; according to Yelena Georgiyevna, he probably had myocarditis a long time ago.

The main criterion in the diagnosis of cardiomyopathy is the selectivity or isolation of myocardial lesions. With regard to clinical symptoms, the ventricle arrhythmia that he suffered was probably the most evident clinical manifestation of cardiomyopathy. Sudden death is not an uncommon outcome of cardiomyopathy, accounting for 43% of all outcomes. There were rumors that foreign cardiologists had recommended the implantation of a pacemaker. However, Yelena Georgiyevna told me that it had been her own idea, which American cardiologists rejected.

In the diagnosis of cardiomyopathy, an analysis of correlations between the autopsy findings and adequate clinical data would be of utmost importance. Unfortunately, in Sakharov's case, the material produced by clinical observations was neither sufficiently rich nor capable of enabling a single interpretation. To some extent, this was his own fault because he had not taken enough care of his health for most of his life. Furthermore, in the last years of his life during his exile in Gorky, any care the local medical establishment might have offered him could be compared to the care a hangman might give to a convict to keep him alive until the day of his execution.

In a post-mortem identification of cardiomyopathy, a histological examination of the myocardium is of crucial importance. However, all the materials needed for this examination had been taken away by forensic officers.

Even after his death, Andrey Dmitrievich has remained a human enigma that is not easy to solve...

My father's notes end here. He never got any information on the results of the histological examination of Sakharov's heart. But in August 1995, several months before my father's death, the newspaper *The Doctor* published an article entitled "Academician Sakharov's Disease," written by the Academician Serov, one of the autopsy participants. He wrote that the histological examination had confirmed the diagnosis of cardiomyopathy (as originally suggested by my father). He also wrote that the cardiomyopathy had not been diagnosed during Sakharov's lifetime. This is not accurate. In January 1997, I got a letter from Yelena Bonner where she wrote that the diagnosis of cardiomyopathy had been suggested by an American cardiologist, Dr. Adolph Hutter, a year before Sakharov's death. Dr. Hutter had examined Sakharov in 1988 at the Massachusetts General Hospital, one of the best in the U.S. He wrote in his conclusions: "Based on the data obtained during the examination, I may say with a high degree of confidence that you have a cardiomyopathy that to some extent has affected both cavities of your heart." Very tactfully, Dr. Hutter suggested that the ineffective therapy prescribed by his Soviet colleagues should be replaced with a different treatment. Unfortunately, Russian doctors did not accept his diagnosis and did not follow his recommendations.

When Yelena Bonner came to visit us after the autopsy, our telephone gave a click and stopped working. It returned to normal the moment she left. Evidently, she was not the only person who was interested in my father's opinion on the cause of Sakharov's sudden death. Powerful electronic eavesdropping devices were probably focused on our dining room where the conversation took place.

My father began the interview by asking her whether she knew anything about the circumstances of Sakharov's birth. She immediately confirmed his hypothesis about Sakharov's birth trauma. Later, in her letter to me, she described this in more detail: *He was delivered without the use of forceps, but the delivery was complicated and he was born with a cephalohematoma.* My father proceeded to list every ailment Andrey Sakharov had suffered during his life, based on the results of the autopsy, and Yelena confirmed every one of his conclusions with growing amazement. I listened, enthralled, even though I was well accustomed to his exceptional professionalism.

In 1997, I asked Yelena Bonner for her endorsement to publish my father's and my notes on Sakharov's autopsy (in Russian). She responded with the friendly letter presented below.

Elena Bonner

Дорогая Наташа!

Конечно же, у меня нет никаких возражений против Вашей публикации. Но мне хотелось бы, чтобы Вы внесли несколько небольших исправлений, если сочтете это возможным.

1) Я не должна была разбудить А.Д. звонком (стр. 2), а просто спустилась к нему, чтобы разбудить.

2) Двери у нас вообще традиционно днем (фактически до ночи) не запирались. Я и сейчас так живу.

3) Щитин в родах не исследовали, но роды были тяжелые и была послеродовая цефало-гематома. (стр. 11)

В письме от 23 мая 1921 г. (т.е. после двух дней — А.Д. родился 21 мая) его дядя Владимир Алексеевич Софиано написал своей крестной: „Роды были вторые по трудности!" Я не знаю, что это означало по тогдашней квалификации, но такой вот документ — письмо — сохранился.

4) Доктор A. Hutter (Mass. General Hosp. Boston) в ноябре 1988 г. поставил А.Д. диагноз кардиомиопатии и (правда, очень сдержанно и тактично) неодобрил применение тех медикаментов, которые назначались А.Д. в Горьком и врачами Академии. Посылаю Вам копию его заключения и буду рада, если Вы ее процитируете в примечаниях.

Спасибо Вам за Ваш труд и доброе отношение

Елена Боннэр

26 июл 1997 г.
Бостон.

P.S. Тот же д-р Hutter уже обследовал его ранее 5 ... и также констатировал, и он признал причины ухудшения.

Translation of Yelena Bonner's letter:

Dear Natasha!

Of course, I have no objections to your publication. I would only prefer to see a couple of minor corrections made, if you agree

1) *I was supposed to simply come downstairs to wake A.D. [Andrey Dmitrievich] up, not call him on the phone (p. 2)*

2) *We never locked our doors during the day and basically until late at night. I'm still living like that.*

3) *He was delivered without the use of forceps, but the delivery was complicated, and he was born with a cephalohematoma (p. 11)*

   Two days after that birth, on May 23, 1921, his uncle, Vladimir Alexeyevich Sofiano, wrote to his godmother: 'The delivery was of second degree in terms of complexity.' I don't know what this might mean, perhaps a reference to some kind of obstetrical ranking used at the time, but there it is — surviving documentary evidence.

4) *Dr. A. Hutter (Mass. General Hosp. Boston) diagnosed A.D. in November 1988 with cardiomyopathy and expressed, albeit in a very restrained and tactful form, his disagreement with the drugs prescribed to A.D. by his local doctors in Gorky and his doctors at the Medical Academy. I am enclosing a copy of his notes and will be grateful if you can quote them in a footnote.*

Many thanks for your work and your friendship.

Yelena Bonner

January 26, 1997

Boston

P.S. Dr. Hutter, who examined A.D. and monitored his heart and consulted with his colleagues, also advised against a pacemaker.

*****

Then there was the farewell ceremony. Despite a bone-chilling frost, tens of thousands of people came to say goodbye to Andrey Sakharov. The line of mourners stretched for at least half a mile and moved forward at a glacial pace. The ceremony was organized by my friends from the *Memorial*. This human-rights organization, the first true grassroots organization in the Soviet Union, had been founded less than a year prior in January 1989, with Andrey Sakharov as one of its co-founders and the chairman. In a display of civic spirit that was very uncommon for the Soviet Union, young men and women went out into the streets, theaters, concert halls, and stadiums in Moscow and other big cities collecting signatures under a petition to build a memorial for victims of Stalin's repressions. The petition was addressed to the 19th (and last) Conference of the Communist Party of the USSR and was accepted. I was part of the *Memorial* from the time of its inception and helped write its bylaws. My membership card bears the number 94 and Andrey Sakharov's own signature.

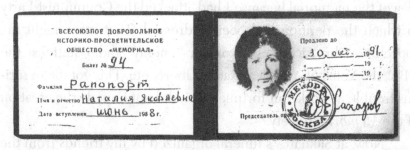

Natalia Rapoport's membership card signed by Andrey Sakharov.

I spoke at the inaugural conference of the *Memorial*, chaired by three prominent writers: Anatoly Rybakov, Mikhail Shatrov, and Yevgeny Yevtushenko. My speech caused something of a stir. Every speaker before me talked about creating a monument to the victims of Stalin's repressions from the 1930s to the 1950s.

Indignantly, I said, "I am shocked at all these proposals to restrict the scope of the memorial to this narrow range. We all know it did not start in the 1930s, nor did it end in the 1950s... Unless we admit that the victims we are talking about today were victims of the totalitarian regime as a whole and not of Stalin alone, we might as well leave room on the memorial stones for our own names."

My words were greeted with dead silence. This may well have been the first time that anyone, speaking from an open podium in the presence of major media from all over the world, had named the real criminal — the Communist Party — and attacked the totalitarian system itself. Then the Sakharovs (who were sitting in the audience, even though I thought they should have been invited up on stage) began to applaud, followed by a few people in the audience. Most kept silent; in those early days of *Perestroika*, the fear still held sway. Then Mikhail Shatrov shouted from the stage that my speech was a provocation aimed at ruining the whole idea of the memorial because I had attacked the Communist Party to which the petition had been addressed. That same night my speech was broadcast by all major "enemy" radio stations: the BBC, the Voice of America, Radio Liberty etc. This got me in serious trouble at work, but fortunately, it did not impede the creation of the *Memorial* society.

Now, at Sakharov's funeral organized by my friends from the *Memorial*, I could not bring myself to go to the head of the line of mourners but stood in line with everyone else. When I finally got to the door, my fellow *Memorial* friends remonstrated with me: "Where have you been? Why did you stay in the line? Everyone is waiting for you!"

And so they were. The rumors had spread like wildfire all over Moscow; people already knew that my father had participated in the autopsy and I had accompanied him. It was widely rumored that Sakharov had been murdered, so everyone wanted to hear what I had to say. I was immediately surrounded by a dense crowd and had to repeat over and over that the pathologists had not found any signs of violent death, that Sakharov had died of cardiac arrest. It was the literal truth, but of course it was not the whole truth. All of us knew that the mistreatment he had endured at the hands of the regime in his last years had killed him just as surely as did those "natural causes" listed in his death certificate.

I stood in the honor guard. It was a great honor. I knew that I was representing my 91-year-old father who, throughout his long life in Russia, had never gone against his conscience, just as Sakharov had never gone against his.

7 Chapter Mischka

Her friends called her Mischka. I met this woman through some mutual friends when, after Stalin's death, she returned to Moscow after spending about two decades in prisons, labor camps, and exile. We quickly became good friends. People told wildly romantic stories about her; those of us who knew Mischka found them easy to believe.

In the early 1920s, Mischka, a Latvian Jew married to a German Communist, acted as a courier for the Communist International, or Comintern — an international Communist organization created by Vladimir Lenin in 1919 that advocated world Communism. By order of the top Bolshevik leadership, Mischka delivered diamonds and other jewels taken from the deposed Romanov dynasty to Communists in England and Germany in order to fund the world revolution. Mischka and her partner sailed in luxury liners and stayed in the best staterooms, playing the part of a free-spending rich couple. Mischka wore expensive clothes and exquisite jewelry, although she didn't dare to display the actual jewels from Romanov's crown. Upon arrival, Mischka would hand all the jewels over to local Party officials. She loved that life. But there was once she and her partner were swindled and robbed by a pair of talented thieves who had somehow gotten wind of the precious cargo they were carrying. This would make a great Hollywood movie; perhaps someday I will describe it in more detail!

After Lenin's death, Stalin infiltrated the Comintern with the Soviet secret police. He used the Comintern as a cover for spies but did not trust its members. In the purges of the 1930s, Stalin arrested and killed one-third of the Comintern staff members. With exquisite cruelty that was so typical of Stalin, those German Communists and antifascists who had fled from Nazi Germany to the Soviet Union were either executed or handed over back to Nazi Germany, an ultimate betrayal.

Mischka was lucky; she was "merely" imprisoned. One day, she told me her story and the truth turned out to be a hundred times more fascinating, romantic and convoluted than the wildest possible fantasy.

Prologue

…The car flew along the autobahn. Signs in German kept flashing by and disappearing, merging into one endless and meaningless sentence. The old man behind the wheel stared ahead. He looked as though he was concentrating on the road, but the woman in the passenger seat next to him knew that he was deeply immersed in his thoughts, and she was worried. From time to time, he glanced over at her with a stunned and incredulous expression on his face, as if he doubted the very fact of her existence. Looking at this silent old couple, a stranger would never guess that the silver Mercedes was speeding them toward a reunion with their stolen youth…

1. The Specter of Communism is Haunting Europe

In the early twenties of what is now the last century, the *Polizeipraesidium* of the city of Berlin married two young Communists: Kurt Muller, a German, and a Latvian Jewish woman whom everybody called Mischka because her real name, Wilhelmina [Magidson], was outlandishly long, like a trail in a jungle, and did not suit her at all. The bride was slender, graceful, and brimming with joy. She looked especially charming in a simple pastel dress with a small bouquet of wild flowers in her hands. This did not escape the attention of an elegant young woman, probably French, who was waiting for the newlyweds outside the *Polizeipraesidium's* door. It appeared that nobody — neither the newlyweds themselves nor their few guests — knew her. They walked outside, got into a car, and drove away to celebrate the wedding at a small restaurant.

The woman took a few steps after them before turning away into an alley, and here we part with her to meet again at a time designated by fate — approximately fifty years later.

Meanwhile, at the restaurant, after a quick toast to the newlyweds' unclouded marital bliss, the guests switched their conversation to politics. The specter of Communism was haunting Europe at the time, generating winds that scattered its young and energetic followers all over the world. One such wind, in 1931, brought our young couple to Moscow where Kurt, who was a natural leader, became Secretary of the Communist International of Young People, or KIM. Mischka worked for the Third Communist International, or Comintern, as a secretary to the prominent leader of the Bulgarian Communist Party, Georgy Dimitrov.

Impulsive and romantic, Kurt did not exactly fit in well with the Soviet leadership circles. Soon he fell out with Stalin, who accused him of "leftist deviation," stripped him of his leadership position, and sent him to be "rehabilitated" by making him serve at a low-level Party cell at a large plant in the city of Gorky. Too proud to accept his demotion, Kurt returned to Germany. Mischka stayed in Moscow for what they thought would be a temporary separation. The year was 1934.

Kurt was horrified with what he found at home. Instead of the civilized, refined countrymen he remembered, the streets were full of screaming hoodlums and marching shopkeepers spouting hateful slogans and brandishing arms adorned with swastikas. And this was the nation that had given the world Beethoven, Heine and Goethe — not to mention, Marx himself?

Kurt's return home from the USSR did not pass unnoticed. Once he ran into a former classmate, now a successful Schutzstaffel (SS) officer, in the street. Kurt's hard-left opinions were well known among his fellow schoolmates. The former friend did not hesitate long before denouncing him, and soon Kurt was arrested.

He did not break down in the Gestapo jail, did not betray his fellow Communists, and was sentenced to six years in solitary confinement.

Mischka's turn came two years later. In 1936, Mischka was arrested in Moscow, together with other Comintern members, when Stalin suppressed the Third International.

And this is how the young Communist couple spent the rest of the 1930s and most of the 1940s: he in a Gestapo prison, she in a Bolshevik one...

When WWII started, Kurt's sentence was extended and he was transferred to the Ziekenhuizen concentration camp. He stayed there until he was released by the British Army in 1945.

After his release, Kurt immediately started searching for Mischka, but all his attempts to find information led him down blind alleys. Rumors about the tragic fate of the Third International's members had reached the West, but Kurt wanted to keep his dream alive and continued waiting in hopes that, by some miracle, Mischka would materialize out of his dreams. But the miracle never happened and Kurt finally came to the bitter conclusion that Mischka had most likely perished.

2. Wives of "Traitors to the Motherland"

And yet she *was* alive… Unlike Kurt, Mischka spent her prison days not in solitary confinement but in a communal cell instead, into which an endless tide brought "wives of traitors to the Motherland" from the outside. Unaware of what was happening outside, Mischka was convinced that she (of course) had been arrested by mistake while those around her were real enemies who had known of their husbands' criminal activities and condoned them. She studied their faces: old and young, pretty and plain, city women and peasants — the NKVD machine did not spare anyone. In her overcrowded prison cell, she talked to no one and kept to herself, as though sentencing herself to solitary confinement. Her arrest had destroyed the last remaining glimmer of hope that she and Kurt would someday be reunited. Her happy, colorful past faded away, replaced by the endless, drab routine of prison life.

One day, the tide brought a pretty young woman to the bunk bed next to Mischka's. The woman had a friendly and intelligent face but looked so sad that Mischka decided to break her silence. They talked. The woman's name was Nyusya Larina (Bukharina).

"Bukharina? Why, how?" It emerged that Nyusya was the wife of Nikolay Bukharin, an Old Bolshevik, one of the founders of the Bolshevik revolution. If Nyusya was there as a "wife of a traitor to the Motherland," why, that meant that Bukharin himself…

"Arrested?!" Mischka was stunned. Bukharin, arrested as a traitor? She and Kurt used to know Bukharin and held him in great esteem. How could *he* be an enemy of the people?

That was the moment of her epiphany. She looked once again at the faces around her. Old and young, pretty and plain, city women and peasants... Were they really all enemies?

This moment of truth saved her sanity, because now she had friends. Most of these friendships blossomed briefly and then died, interrupted by the prison reshufflings. Fortunately for Mischka, she and Nyusya Bukharina were able to stay together for almost the entire duration of their prison time; their prison transit routes ran side by side...

Eventually, Mischka was sentenced to eight years in a maximum-security labor camp and was sent to Ust'-Vym' Lag, a remote place in the Far North of Russia. This tiny woman, whose body could hardly be seen under the oversized quilted jacket they gave her in camp, was assigned to log trees in the taiga. The diminutive Mischka did not make a good logger. Besides, she constantly got into trouble. It would not be hard to predict how it would have ended had she not met Naum.

3. Naum

Naum Slavutsky was not yet twenty when he was arrested. He was serving in the Soviet Army at the time of his arrest. He was naïve and had an inquisitive mind. During a political orientation class, he was careless enough to ask the wrong question about Trotskyism. His answer was an eight-year sentence in the camps. He was arrested on the last scheduled day of his Army service and sent to Ust'-Vym' Lag.

Naum was short and stocky but well-built, strong, and very smart. Despite his youth, he was assigned as a supervisor over Mischka's logging site. There they met and fell in love.

Naum's term ended before Mischka's but he did not leave the area. Where would he have gone anyway? His release papers carried the infamous code of "minus thirty-nine." That was not a reference to prevailing winter temperatures (in Celsius) in Ust'-Vym' Lag; it meant that the bearer is denied residency privileges in the thirty-nine largest cities of his vast Motherland. Waiting for Mischka's release, Naum rented a log cabin near the camp and found a job as a freedman contractor working for the camp administration. In his new position, he managed to convince the camp authorities to have Mischka reassigned to somewhat easier labor. It saved her life.

Mischka's term ended in 1944 but nothing further was said about her release. And then a miracle happened. Mischka's former boss at the Third Comintern, Georgy Dimitrov, who had inexplicably avoided arrest and still occupied a high position in the Communist hierarchy, tracked her down, petitioned for her, and in 1946, granted her a "work release." It required her to check in daily at the camp commandant's office, but now she was finally allowed to reside outside the barbed wire.

... Twelve years had passed since Mischka last heard any news about Kurt. To inquire was dangerous and useless. Besides, she was convinced that Kurt could not be alive — there was little chance that he could have survived the Nazi meatgrinder. So Mischka moved in with Naum and later married him and took his name. They lived in a log cabin near the camp and both worked as contract camp staff.

... The winter of 1948 was especially severe. One day, Mischka caught a bad cold and did not report to work. Suddenly, she felt inexplicable anxiety. Pacing feverishly around the small room, she grabbed the power cord of a radio loudspeaker and plugged it in, her hand shaking. Almost immediately she heard the announcer's words:

"...His deputy Kurt Muller said..."

But what Kurt Muller said, neither we nor the deeply shaken Mischka will ever know. Mischka missed the rest of the statement, brought to her godforsaken camp in the Far North of Russia by that beat-up old radio. While she was trying to pull herself together, the rest of the statement got lost amidst the usual deluge of news about the growing prosperity of the Soviet people.

She did, however, grasp that Kurt was alive — and not merely alive but obviously holding a high position. Otherwise, why would the Soviet radio quote his statement?

In fact, at that time Kurt was Deputy General Secretary of the West German Communist Party and a member of the Bundestag.

That was how Mischka came to the realization that she was now technically a polyandrist. However, she had no way of getting in touch with Kurt. It also appeared easier and less dangerous to simply cross out and forget her past life, especially since after that radio incident, Kurt seemed to disappear from the surface of the Earth again. At least, Mischka never again heard anything about him on the radio.

4. Kurt

The reader may recall that in the beginning of 1945 Kurt was released from a Nazi concentration camp by the British Army. After the ten years he had spent in a Nazi prison, he came out an even more fervent Communist than before. He joined the Adenauer government as a representative of the West German Communist Party. Once Kurt was back in a high position, he was once again noticed by Stalin, and the Soviet Generalissimo never forgot nor forgave.

In 1951, a Congress of the East German Communist Party took place in East Berlin. On Stalin's instructions, the Eastern Communists invited their West German Party comrade over for a gathering, where he was kidnapped by East German special agents. The Bundestag lodged an official protest, but despite a growing political scandal, the East Germans transferred Kurt to Moscow where he was locked up in the infamous Vladimirskaya Central Prison, or *Vladimirka*. Reflecting his exquisite cruelty, Stalin placed him in the same cell with Nazi generals taken as prisoners of war during WWII. So after spending a decade imprisoned by the Nazis, now, due to a brilliant twist in Stalin's screenplay, Kurt Muller was sharing a cell with them in a Communist prison. The Soviet regime delighted in putting the hunters and their prey into the same cage...

And so, for the first time in twenty years, Kurt and Mischka found themselves on the same side of the Iron Curtain where they could, one day, run into each other again on one of the many islands of the Gulag Archipelago. But neither of them had any premonition of that...

5. 1956 in Moscow

Stalin's death on March 5, 1953 was secretly celebrated by millions. Then came the year of 1956 which was filled with surprises — beginning with Nikita Khrushchev's unprecedented speech openly denouncing Stalin's crimes. During this period which later came to be known as a "thaw," Mischka and Naum were rehabilitated. They returned to Moscow and settled in a small apartment along Profsoyuznaya Street. Unbeknownst to them, Kurt was at that time still in Vladimirskaya prison, only a hundred kilometers away...

Still as charming and energetic as ever and a wonderful storyteller, Mischka quickly won over Moscow's intelligentsia circles. Many writers, artists, and actors she met during that time became her friends for life. She became involved with the dissidents and human rights activists and participated in *samizdat*. Such prominent writers as Alexander Solzhenitsyn and Lev Kopelev, just to name a couple, were among the Slavutskys' friends. Soon the small apartment on Profsoyuznaya Street turned into a salon for former political prisoners and later a center for the opposition. Mischka confidently navigated her small ship through the raging waters of the "thaw."

Meanwhile, Khrushchev and Adenauer signed an agreement guaranteeing the return of German prisoners of war. The fact that Kurt shared a cell with Nazi generals suddenly became an advantage: by mistake, he was included in the list of German POWs and was shipped directly from Vladimirskaya Prison to Germany. But he and Mischka never heard anything about each other and hence they did not meet…

The Soviet Communists managed to do what the Gestapo failed to accomplish in ten years: upon his return to Germany, Kurt Muller immediately resigned from the Communist Party.

… One day, the renowned German writer Heinrich Böll came to Moscow. In the mid-1960s he was in great favor with the Soviets, who considered him a progressive writer. Somebody brought him to see Mischka and she told him her story.

"Kurt is alive," said an astonished Böll. "He was imprisoned, first by the Nazis and then by your people. He was convinced that you had died. He got married just recently."

Soon after Böll's visit, Mischka received a postcard from Kurt, the first tiny piece of news after thirty years of separation. His experience in Soviet prison taught him that a postcard had a better chance of reaching the addressee than a sealed letter did. The message was laconic: *"If you want to learn more about me, find a man in Moscow named Vassily Vassilievich Parin."*

"My little Kurt, still a hopeless romantic," commented Mischka. "Easy for him to say: find a man named Parin! It's like finding a needle in a haystack…"

But here, yet another miracle happened.

"There was a pediatrician who used to work at our clinic and her last name was Parina," said one of Mischka's friends. "She resigned recently. I didn't know her closely, but I will try to find out; she may be related to your Parin."

The very next day, Mischka had the address and telephone number of Vassily Vassilievich Parin.

Mischka guessed that this Parin's association with Kurt must have had something to do with his time in Vladimirskaya prison. She did not use the telephone; people did not discuss things like that over the phone in the 1960s. She simply went to the address on Begovaya Street.

The doorbell was answered by a boy of about fourteen. He opened the door just a crack. Mischka thought she saw a door chain.

"Who do you need to see?"

"Excuse me, may I see Vassily Vassilievich Parin?"

"Papa is not home."

"When is he going to be back?"

"In an hour."

An hour and a half later, after pacing up and down Begovaya Street, Mischka rang the bell again. This time an older boy looked out through the crack:

"Papa does not see people at home."

"Does not see people at home…" Mischka was confused. *"Who is he? A doctor? A lawyer?"* she thought to herself. But aloud, she said:

"This is a personal matter. I need to see him."

At that moment, a tall, regal-looking man with an intelligent face appeared in the corridor behind the boy. He opened the door wide; it turned out there was no chain. He looked at Mischka in what she thought was a somewhat aloof and guarded manner and asked:

"How can I help you?"

The curious faces of the two boys with whom Mischka had spoken were peeking out from behind the man's back. She was not sure what the children might know about their father's past and asked if she could talk to the man privately.

The man shrugged coldly and showed her into his study. Never in her life had Mischka seen such a spacious and luxurious study, all paneled in wood. This was not an interior decorating style used in the camp barracks or log cabins… She felt embarrassed and thought: *"I must have made a mistake, this must be the wrong Parin."*

The formidable man repeated impatiently:

"So how can I help you?"

Her tongue practically cleaving to the roof of her dry mouth, Mischka asked hesitantly:

"Does the name Kurt Muller mean anything to you?"

"Mischka?!"

It was as if two bright lights were switched on in the eyes of this forbidding man. Scooping her up in his arms, Parin waltzed around the study, heedless of the danger to his expensive furniture, saying in a sing-song voice:

"Mischka! Mischka! Mischka! How did I not recognize you right away? There were so many days and nights when Kurt spoke of nothing but you! I thought I would recognize you at once if I saw you, but I didn't!"

"You haven't changed at all," said Parin, who had never seen Mischka before. "Kurt thought that you were dead. What a joy that you are alive! Well, tell me everything!"

"No, you first."

Of course, he was the *right* Parin. As we already know, back in 1947, Dr. Parin had been put in the terrible Vladimirskaya prison in connection with the case of the anti-cancer vaccine known as *KR*. He had spent many years in the same cell with Kurt. The two of them became close friends. They had plenty of time to talk... Neither of them paid any attention to their other cellmates, the German generals.

Parin spoke for several hours, telling Mischka about Kurt: the Gestapo, the solitary confinement, the Nazi concentration camp, and how, after his release, Kurt had looked for her for a long time before deciding, in despair, that she was no longer alive... He told her about how Kurt was invited to East Germany and kidnapped, and how he spent the long years in Vladimirskaya Prison...

Then Mischka told Parin her story, walking him through her life day by day, from the Comintern to prison, from prison to labor camp. Finally, she told him about Naum.

"Please tell me what I can do for you," Parin pleaded. "There's a lot I can do!"

"I don't need anything," Mischka answered firmly. Despite Parin's repeated requests, she did not give him her address or telephone number. She did not even give him her new married name. She understood that Parin held a very high position — his apartment and study spoke for themselves — and she did not want him to jeopardize himself and his family by associating with her…

Mischka's intuition about Parin's position in the Soviet hierarchy was correct. Academician Vassily Vassilievich Parin was, at that time, the director of the State Institute of Medical and Biological Problems and the Academician Secretary of the Academy of Medical Sciences of the USSR.

6. Victory Day

After Böll's visit, Mischka and Kurt exchanged occasional postcards. They knew that their correspondence was read by the authorities, so they only sent birthday and holiday greetings with trivial messages. Between their last meeting and their first postcard lay an eternity. Forty tragic years (the total combined time the two of them spent in concentration camps) had been stolen from them. They both had new families and new lives. They certainly had a lot to talk about, but for that they needed to meet, and that was far more than they could ever hope for. After marrying Naum, Mischka had become a Soviet citizen and, naturally, was not allowed to travel abroad. After his experience in Vladimirskaya prison, Kurt would never dream of setting foot on Soviet soil again. And so their lives continued in parallel, worlds apart, with no indication that their paths would ever cross again. Until suddenly, in 1975, Mischka received a strange postcard.

"Suddenly" is one of the colors life uses to brighten up our routine. Each life has its own palette — some people's palettes have more colors on them than others. Mischka's contained the whole spectrum.

So it was that one day Mischka received a strange postcard from Paris. It was written in French and signed "M. Raboteur."

"I cannot even tell whether it was written by a man or a woman," complained Mischka.

The unknown correspondent wrote that he or she would be visiting Moscow to attend the Red Square parade celebrating the thirtieth anniversary of the Soviet victory over the Nazis. The sender wrote that they needed to meet and asked Mischka if she could be at home on the day of the parade and wait for a telephone call.

The name Raboteur was vaguely familiar to Mischka. It seemed to belong to a long-forgotten past that no longer felt real, but she could not recall any details.

On Victory Day, she stayed at home. Half an hour after the end of the parade on Red Square, the telephone rang.

"I am Marie Raboteur," said a woman with a slightly husky voice, in French. "I will be waiting for you in an hour in front of the National Hotel."

"Fine, but how will we recognize each other?"

"Oh, don't worry, I will recognize *you*."

Was it Mischka's imagination… or did she actually hear a trace of bitter sarcasm in the woman's voice?

An hour later, an intrigued Mischka approached the National Hotel. An unfamiliar, aged but elegant woman walked toward her. Mischka could swear that she had never seen her before — but you, my reader, may have already recalled the young French woman who had waited outside the Berlin *Polizeipraesidium*'s office during Mischka's wedding ceremony, more than forty years earlier!

"I am Marie Raboteur," said the woman. "Let's go up to my room; we need to talk."

They went up to Marie's hotel room. There, Marie further surprised Mischka by her familiarity with Mischka's past. Mischka did not have the slightest idea who the woman was but felt too embarrassed to ask because the woman behaved as if Mischka was supposed to know her. She also clearly enjoyed Mischka's confusion. The situation was becoming awkward when Mischka came upon a brilliant idea: she would invite Marie to her house to meet Naum. He certainly had never met her, so it would be natural if he asked a few questions.

The woman agreed at once, as if she had been waiting for this invitation. But at home, after Naum's careful questions failed to shed any light on the mysterious visitor, Marie finally decided that she had mystified them enough and asked if she could talk to Mischka privately.

7. Marie Raboteur's Story

Many years ago before her marriage to Kurt, Mischka met a young French Communist, Auguste Raboteur, at one of the Communist meetings in Paris and he fell in love with her. He sent her flowers from all over the world — Europe, Asia, North and South America, everywhere his Party assignments took him. Auguste was prepared to leave his beautiful, loving wife Marie for Mischka. Mischka did not encourage the affair. She did not want to build her happiness upon someone else's tragedy, and besides, by that time, she had already met Kurt.

"I knew that Auguste was madly in love with you," Marie told Mischka. "Once, I read about you in his diary. But never mind the diary. You did not know me, but I followed you everywhere, studied the way you walked, talked, dressed... I was trying to understand what it was about you that won over Auguste's heart...

Guess who was the happiest person on your wedding day when you married Kurt? You think it was you? No, my dear, it was me. I came all the way to Berlin and followed you to the *Poli-zeipraesidium*. I waited outside until you left and then went off to celebrate by myself at a fancy restaurant.

Auguste suffered terribly when you got married. I pretended that I did not notice and did not know the reason. Then you and Kurt went to the USSR. I hoped that time and distance would cure Auguste, but he continued tracking all the twists and turns of your life as best as he could. We knew that Kurt fell out with Stalin and returned to Germany, was arrested by the Gestapo and disappeared, and that you remained in Moscow. And then you disappeared, too. The next time he found your trace was only in the late '50s, when you returned from the Gulag.

After your disappearance at the end of the '30s, the war started, and Auguste, of course, went to Spain to fight. He was captured by the Francoists and sentenced to death, but then he managed to escape. He returned to France with fake documents and we joined the Resistance. This brought us very close. I was happy.

Then he was arrested again, this time by the German fascists. He ended up in a German concentration camp but survived due to his fake documents. I took his place and became a leader in the French women's Resistance movement.

When the war ended, I was elected to the French Senate. Auguste was very proud of me. Those were our happiest years.

But one day, his doctor called me and asked me to see him. He told me that Auguste had liver cancer, and that he had not told him about it. He suggested that I take Auguste to the country house where he would have a lot of fresh air. He warned me that Auguste would be in terrible pain. He gave me some drugs to inject when the pain started. Then he gave me one more vial. 'The day will come,' he said, 'when these drugs no longer help. For this day, here is one last vial. I know you and I am sure you will not use it without ultimate need.'

We moved out to the country. The pain started pretty soon and I started giving him the shots. Of course, he knew about his diagnosis, but we did not speak about it. He lost a lot of weight. One day the shot did not help. I suggested that I could give him another shot. He declined:

'I will manage,' he said. 'I have looked into the eyes of death too many times. I don't need help with this. You better just bring me a bottle of wine.'"

I did, and suddenly it was all right. We did not have to pretend any longer. I opened a bottle of wine and we talked for a long time. Auguste tried to prepare me for my future life without him. And then he said:

'Marie, I have to tell you something. All my life, I have loved another woman.'

I said: 'I know.'

'Marie, I have a great favor to ask. Find Mischka. She now lives in Moscow and her last name is Slavutskaya. Tell her about me. It is important to me that she knows about my life and that it leaves at least some mark in hers.'

I promised. By morning, he was gone.

Several months passed and suddenly, as leader of the Women's Resistance, I received an invitation to attend the Red Square parade in Moscow. It felt like a sign from the beyond, as though this was Auguste reminding me about my promise. I managed to find your address and telephone number — and here I am."

Marie left the next day. Soon after her departure, Mischka received a second postcard from Paris. "*How silly of me,*" Marie wrote, "*Why did I not think of inviting you? Just imagine how happy Auguste would be if you could visit his house, walk on the same floor and breathe the same air!"*

"Why, Marie," Mischka responded, "have you forgotten where I live? Who is going to let me go?"

"Am I not a leader of the Women's Resistance movement?" Marie replied.

And one month later, the telephone rang in Mischka's apartment:

"We are calling from the office of Leonid Ilyich Brezhnev. Your foreign passport is ready for your trip to France. You may go to the OVIR[1] to pick it up."

At the OVIR, an officer admonished Mishka:

"Your passport is valid for France *only*. Don't even think of visiting other countries."

"I won't," said Mischka.

8. The Train to Paris

The train from Moscow to Paris makes a fifteen-minute stopover in Böll's city of Cologne. Mischka called Böll.

"I am going on an unexpected trip to Paris and stopping over in Cologne. Perhaps we can meet on the platform?"

"Of course!" said Böll.

He was right there when the train stopped. In front of the stunned passengers he literally "kidnapped" Mischka, lifted her up in his arms, took her off the train, and did not let her go until the train had left.

Böll brought Mischka to his country house. They had a glass of wine.

---

[1] The OVIR was the Russian counterpart to the American Immigration and Naturalization service.

"This room is for you," Böll said. "The last person to sleep in this bed was Alexander Solzhenitsyn. Do you see the shed with no roof? It collapsed when reporters from all over the world climbed on top of it when I brought Solzhenitsyn here from the airport after he was expelled from the Soviet Union. I am not fixing the shed on purpose; it stands there as a monument to those days."

"You need some sleep," Böll suddenly interrupted himself. "You've got a long day ahead of you tomorrow."

The next morning, an enormous bouquet of Mischka's favorite wild flowers entered her room in Heinrich Böll's house. Behind the flowers was Mischka's first husband, Kurt Muller.

"Mischka, what did you feel? Please tell me what you felt at that moment?" I begged.

"Nothing," Mischka answered. "Too many years had passed; our lives had been too different. He was a stranger..."

Kurt brought Mischka to his home. The door was opened by a younger looking woman — Kurt's wife. She welcomed Mischka like a dear friend, hugged and kissed her. Kurt watched his wife with tenderness and gratitude; it was clear that he was happy in his second marriage. But when they entered the house, Mischka froze in place. Looking down upon her from every wall were photographs of their youth: the young and beautiful Mischka, laughing and waving her hand at Kurt in Paris, Berlin, Moscow. She had completely forgotten about these pictures; she had even forgotten what she herself had looked like when she was young. She had saved nothing from that past life — not a shred of paper, nothing in her heart. But Kurt had.

"You should take down these photos," Mischka said to Kurt. "It must be very hard on your wife. It looks as if there are three people living in this house: you, your wife, and my shadow."

"No need," Kurt's wife said. "It won't change anything. You are always with him. I have learned to accept and love you…"

…The car flew along the autobahn. Signs in German kept flashing by and disappearing, merging into one endless and meaningless sentence. The old man behind the wheel stared ahead. He looked as though he was concentrating on the road, but the woman in the passenger seat next to him knew that he was deeply immersed in his thoughts, and she was worried. From time to time, he glanced over at her with a stunned and incredulous expression on his face, as if he doubted the very fact of her existence. Looking at this silent old couple, a stranger would never guess that the silver Mercedes was speeding them toward a reunion with their stolen youth…

Epilogue

As soon as the Iron Curtain lifted, Mischka and Naum moved to Germany. Böll got them into a retirement home where they had a little apartment to themselves, free healthcare, and were generally taken care of. I came to visit them twice; they looked happy. Mischka was over a hundred years old when she passed away. She was sick during her last years, and Naum took care of her faithfully. She was his life; he died less than a year after her passing.

8 The Kanel Family and the Secrets of the Kremlin Hospital

My parents kept a photograph that I long thought was a postcard. It showed a beautiful young woman dressed in 1930s fashion standing beside an athletic young man against the background of a Crimean landscape, looking like two movie stars. In the same old photo album, I also saw her photograph with my father against the same background. I later learned that it was a close friend of my parents', Nadezhda Veniaminovna Kanel (to her friends, "Dynochka"). She and her second husband, Adolph Slomyansky,

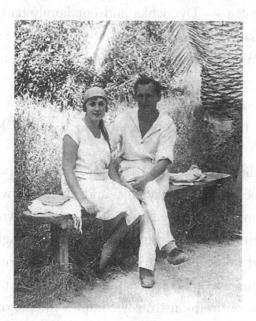

Dynochka Kanel and Yakov Rapoport in Crimea in 1933.

were often guests in our house. In the magnificent "choir" of intellectuals that used to grace my parents' hospitable table, Adolph Slomyansky was one of the leading voices. He was a witty storyteller, a discriminating connoisseur of music, art, and history, a good singer, and an extraordinarily handsome man.

They came into my life during the early days of Khrushchev's thaw, when Dynochka was released from prison where she had spent more than a decade. Adolph faithfully waited for her all those years.

Dynochka was the daughter of Alexandra Yulianovna Kanel, Head Doctor of the Kremlin hospital at the time of the death of Stalin's wife, Nadezhda Alliluyeva. Like her mother, indeed like anyone who had been connected even slightly with Alliluyeva's death — people who knew too much, those who knew something, or simply curious strangers who were foolish enough to have asked questions about it — Dynochka and her family had been swept away in its wake.

Alexandra Yulianovna Kanel died under strange circumstances. Her daughters Dynochka and Lyalya (Yulia) were arrested. Lyalya was executed in prison; Dynochka survived, by sheer chance, two prison sentences from 1939 to 1945 and from 1948 to 1953.

Adolph died in the mid-1980s. Many of my parents' other friends died before him. Dynochka and my father were "the last of the Mohicans." When my father died in 1996, Dynochka could not bring herself to attend his funeral, but that night she came to see me and told me her story. Although I had heard most of it before in bits and pieces, she put it all together for me that evening — the entire monstrously complex mosaic of people and events associated with the death of Stalin's wife. Dynochka had an outstanding memory and a crystal-clear mind. I recorded her story and donated the tape to the Hoover Institution Archives.

1. Stalin's Wife Nadezhda Alliluyeva Dies at Thirty-One

In the early morning of November 9, 1932, Nadezhda Alliluyeva, Joseph Stalin's second wife, was found dead in her room with a pistol wound at her temple. She was thirty-one.

The official announcement stated that her death had been "sudden and untimely"[1] but gave no further details. This cryptic announcement stirred up a great deal of speculation, especially since she had marched in a parade just the day before and had been seen by thousands of people. A few facts soon leaked out: Alliluyeva had attended a party with Stalin after the parade but left early after a quarrel with her husband and was found dead the next morning.

What was the cause of her sudden death? Stalin ordered the NKVD to circulate an unofficial and implausible report that she had died of acute appendicitis.

Because the cause of Alliluyeva's death was never officially disclosed, it gave rise to a multitude of conflicting rumors: maybe she had taken an overdose of sleeping pills, or maybe she had shot herself in a fit of jealousy over Stalin's philandering (most rumors implicated a Rosa Kaganovich, allegedly a sister of Stalin's closest henchman Lazar Kaganovich, as the major object of Alliluyeva's jealousy). Still others, never uttered above a whisper, insisted that Stalin had strangled her in the bathroom, or that he had shot her

---

[1] Interestingly, the announcement of Alliluyeva's death in the official Soviet newspaper *Pravda* was printed immediately above the announcement of Franklin Delano Roosevelt's victory in the U.S. presidential election.

himself. Many of these rumors, some very persistent, reached the West and were reported by reputable media even though most contained not an ounce of truth.

Clearly determined to never let the truth about his wife's death come to light, Stalin pursued and killed anyone who was even slightly connected to the events of the tragic night of November 8, 1932.

2. The Story of Alexandra Yulianovna Kanel

On the night of November 9, 1932, Alexandra Yulianovna Kanel came home from work and told her daughters, Dynochka and Lyalya: "Last night Nadezhda Alliluyeva killed herself."

Alexandra Kanel was the Head Doctor of the Kremlin Hospital where she treated many Kremlin wives. On the morning of November 9, she set off on her usual rounds. Her first patient that day was the wife of Vyacheslav Molotov, Polina Zhemchuzhina.[2] Kanel found Polina and Molotov in a very troubled state. Molotov said, "Last night, Alliluyeva killed herself." Alexandra asked, "Can I tell people that she committed suicide?" And Molotov answered, "Yes, of course." This was the version of events that Alexandra told her daughters later that night.

After her conversation with the Molotovs, Alexandra went to see her other patient, Olga Davidovna Kameneva. Olga's husband, Lev Kamenev, was the leader of the opposition and had already been sent by Stalin into internal exile. The rest of his family had been evicted from the Kremlin and were living in an apartment in Neglinnaya street, within walking distance of the Kremlin. The

---

[2] The names of the high-ranking Russian politicians mentioned in these stories, although known to historians, may be less familiar to the general reader. Please see a short glossary of their names and positions at the end of the book.

death of Alliluyeva was sensational news, and Kanel told Olga Kameneva that Alliluyeva had committed suicide. Kameneva immediately wrote her exiled husband about it.

Olga Kameneva was Kanel's last patient that day. Leaving her, she went to the Kremlin Hospital. But during those few hours that had passed since Alliluyeva's death, Stalin had invented his own version of the cause of her sudden passing. At 2 pm, two men, Abrosov and Pogosyantz, came into Alexandra Kanel's office. Although styled as doctors, they were really NKVD inspectors assigned to the Kremlin Hospital, presumably to make sure that those patients whom Stalin wanted dead did not survive.

These "doctors" handed Kanel a death certificate stating that Alliluyeva had died of acute appendicitis and ordered her to sign it. Now, dozens of people had seen Alliluyeva the night before at a dinner party at Marshal Voroshilov's home, and even in Russia, nobody dies of appendicitis in such a few short hours. Kanel protested, "I cannot sign this death certificate; I haven't even seen the body." They kept pressing her to sign but she adamantly refused, not realizing that her refusal was tantamount to signing her own death sentence.

The two men approached two other eminent Kremlin doctors, Dr. Lev Levin and Dr. Dmitry Pletnyov, who likewise refused to sign the falsified certificate. Eventually, Abrosov and Pogosyantz did find some other, more compliant doctors who signed the death certificate stating that Alliluyeva had died of appendicitis.

Stalin never forgot or forgave those who had defied his orders and he knew how to wait, carefully choosing the timing of his revenge. In the late 1930s, major Russian newspapers suddenly announced that Dr. Pletnyov (who was then over seventy) had attacked a young patient of his "in a fit of wild passion" and attempted to rape her. The utter absurdity of this accusation did not stop the prosecution. Dr. Pletnyov was arrested and tortured before dying in prison. Dr. Levin suffered a similar fate (minus the accusation of raping a patient); he also died in prison.

Alexandra Kanel was relieved of her duties as Head Doctor of the Kremlin Hospital in 1935, although she kept her position as a regular doctor at the Hospital and continued seeing patients. She looked very depressed. Once Dynochka asked her, "Mom, why don't you just resign?" She answered, "I can't. They will never let me go..."

Alexandra Kanel died suddenly under strange circumstances. In February 1936, she returned from work with a slight cold. It was nothing serious; she did not even stay in bed. They had guests over that night: Dynochka's sister, Lyalya; Lyalya's husband, Severin Veinberg; and Nicolai Villiam-Vilmont, a poet and a renowned literary translator from Germany. He later helped Dynochka to reconstruct the events of that evening.

Unexpectedly, Lev Kamenev's son, Yura, then 15 years old, arrived from the town of Gorky where he was living with his mother who had since been exiled there. Yura Kamenev said that he needed to talk to Alexandra Yulianovna. They went into her study and stayed there for less than ten minutes. Yura came out and left right away. When Alexandra came out of her study, she looked terrible; her face was white and her eyes were unmoving, as if she had suddenly become blind. Dynochka asked, "Mom, what happened? What's wrong?" She responded vaguely, "Olga Davidovna. She is in exile. Alone." Dynochka objected, "Why? She is not alone. She has Yura. She even has a job there. There's no reason to be so upset about it. Why are you so worried?" Alexandra Yulianovna uttered a strange phrase, "Olga Davidovna. The long-suffering Job," and went into her bedroom.

The next morning, Dynochka found her mother unconscious. The family called in Kremlin doctors, who performed a spinal tap and made a diagnosis of streptococcal meningitis. On February 8, 1936 — two days after Yura Kamenev's visit — Alexandra Kanel died without regaining consciousness.

Was her death connected with Yura's visit? Five years later, Dynochka learned some new information when she found herself sharing a prison cell in the city of Oryol with Olga Kameneva, Yura's mother.

Dynochka was arrested during the Great Purges of the 1930s along with her sister Lyalya; Lyalya's husband, Severin Veinberg; Olga Kameneva; and many, many others with ties to, or knowledge (however slight) of, Alliluyeva's death. Most of them were eventually executed. Dynochka was among the very few who survived; she was saved by pure miracle, as will be described later.

...Dynochka arrived at the Oryol prison on June 14, 1941, a week before Hitler invaded the Soviet Union in what would become known in Russia as the "Great Patriotic War." At first, she shared a cell with a very nice woman by the name of Tamara Grin. They got along well, which was a small mercy as strained relationships between cellmates could be an additional source of torment for people sentenced to spend long years together. Both Dynochka and Tamara Grin had five-year sentences, which was considered light in those days. They were together for three months until a stray bullet flew through their window in September and they were moved one floor down and separated. Dynochka entered her new cell and saw Olga Kameneva down on her knees washing the floor. There was another female prisoner in the cell who, like Olga Kameneva, had been sentenced to 25 years in prison (although Olga Kameneva would not be allowed to serve out her sentence: she would be executed a month later, in October 1941).

This encounter was less of a coincidence than it might seem. In Russia's many prisons — those metaphorical islands of the Gulag Archipelago — prisoners were constantly shuffled around like cards in a pack. Some were executed, freeing up space for others. Some were transferred to prisons in different cities and some were just moved to different cells in the same prison. Because people tended to be arrested in groups revolving around some kind of commonality, such as blood or marriage ties, shared friendship or occupation (e.g., archeologists or engineers, politicians or writers), it was not unusual for prisoners to find themselves thrown together with their friends or relatives during this shuffling process.

Olga Kameneva was extremely glad to see Dynochka. Dynochka and her sister Lyalya had previously resented Olga, seeing her as a rival for their mother's time and attention. But now, five years after her mother's death, Dynochka listened with intense attention to Olga Kameneva's story.

Kameneva revealed that she had been very, very fond of Dynochka's mother. She had even sent her son Yura from Gorky to Moscow specifically to warn Alexandra Yulianovna that during Kameneva's first arrest in Moscow, the only person her interrogators questioned her about had been Alexandra Kanel: Why did she say that Alliluyeva had committed suicide? What were her exact words? How did Alexandra know it was a suicide? Why did Kameneva write about it to her husband? *etc., etc.*

"Apparently," Dynochka later said to me, "Mama realized from Yura's message that she was doomed. If the diagnosis of meningitis was correct, the stress probably upset her blood-brain barrier, thus allowing the streptococci to penetrate into her brain which then killed her. That is how I would explain her sudden death. It did not look like a direct murder." Dynochka was a microbiologist; her explanation was her best professional judgment.

Although I respect her judgment, I believe there are other possibilities. Upon realizing that she was doomed, Alexandra Kanel may have taken an overdose of sleeping pills to kill herself in order to avoid arrest and torture. And those Kremlin doctors who visited her may have made sure that she would never wake up...

Stalin had ample reasons to eliminate Alexandra Kanel. He hated her for refusing to sign a false statement about Alliluyeva's death and for her friendship with Molotov's wife, Polina Zhemchuzhina, whom he also hated. And Alexandra simply knew too much. But whether she had committed suicide or had really died from meningitis is something we will never know for sure.

3. The Death Camp at the Kremlin Hospital

"I now understand," Dynochka told me, "that Mama knew about the horrors that were going on in the Kremlin Hospital, but of course she did not say anything to us. Actually, she did tell us once about the strange death of Dmitry Kursky, the People's Commissar for Justice, but apparently at that time she still had no inkling of the criminal activities taking place in the Kremlin Hospital."

Kursky died in 1932, the same year that Nadezhda Alliluyeva died. There had been some sort of falling out between Kursky and Stalin, and in 1928, Kursky was sent to Italy as an ambassador, which was then a sign of disgrace. Kursky spent several years in Italy and was very happy there. But in 1932, he was recalled to Moscow under the pretext that he needed to be hospitalized for medical treatment. He was surprised, protesting that he felt fine. The Kremlin "doctors" told him that he had to be examined and receive treatment for diabetes, prior to being reassigned to a very important mission. So he was admitted to the Kremlin hospital, and two days later he was dead.

Alexandra Kanel had known Kursky and his wife Anna for decades and had even been their family doctor for a period of time. After Kursky's death, Anna Kursky burst into her office and started screaming at her: "You killed my husband! He was in perfect health! You killed him!" Alexandra told her daughters at the time that she was terribly offended by Anna Kursky's behavior, but she also began to suspect that Kursky had indeed been killed at the Hospital.

This was not an isolated incident. In 1925, Mikhail Frunze, the highly popular People's Commissar for Military and Naval Affairs, died under somewhat similar circumstances. Frunze, who had held his post for a mere ten months, disagreed with Stalin on certain matters of policy, and Stalin did not trust him. Frunze's political heterodoxy and his popularity killed him: Stalin did not tolerate popular politicians, especially those who held divergent views.

A lot of information on Frunze's death has since come to light. In 1925, he was hospitalized after a flare-up of his chronic ulcers. On Stalin's demand, the Politburo passed the resolution that he had to undergo surgery. Frunze himself, as well as his attending doctors — Alexandra Kanel and Dr. Rozanov, a prominent surgeon — all protested against the surgery. Frunze wrote to his wife: "At present I am feeling absolutely healthy, and it seems ridiculous to even think about surgery, much less go through with one. Nevertheless, Party representatives demand it." Frunze gave in and agreed to the surgery. Since Dr. Rozanov was against it, another surgeon, Dr. Grekov, was specially summoned from Leningrad. Grekov and Rozanov performed the surgery together with the assistance of Dr. Martynov. During the surgery, the anesthesiologist, Dr. Ochkin, gave Frunze a massive overdose of chloroform. The next day, Frunze was on his deathbed.

Every one of the doctors that had been present during the surgery was later killed, at one time or another. Stalin liked to wait for just the right moment.

There were undoubtedly many other cases of medical homicide at the Kremlin Hospital. The two cases described above took place during Alexandra Kanel's lifetime and have been well documented.

4. Lyalya's Story

In May 1939, Stalin's chief of secret police, Lavrenty Beria, arrested Alexandra Kanel's daughters, Dynochka and Lyalya, both charming and accomplished young women. Dynochka, 35, was a microbiologist; Lyalya, 34, had a Ph.D. in Endocrinology.

At the time of their arrest, Beria, on Stalin's orders, was building a case against Polina Zhemchuzhina, Vyacheslav Molotov's wife. Zhemchuzhina had been a close friend of Stalin's late wife Nadezhda Alliluyeva; Stalin suspected that she knew too much and hated her. He wanted signed confessions from Zhemchuzhina's friends and associates implicating her in espionage. I have never understood why Stalin, a ruler wielding absolute power, should feel the need to build a façade of legality around his butcheries; perhaps he wanted to preserve his image to the West or future generations. In any event, he spared no effort trying to force his victims to confess to crimes they had not committed.

Lyalya Kanel and her husband Severin Veinberg were close friends of Molotov and Zhemchuzhina's. After the sudden death of Lyalya's mother Alexandra Kanel, Molotov organized a trip abroad for Lyalya and Severin. The couple spent two months abroad. Because Severin had relatives in Paris and in Palestine, they were expected to get monetary support from them. Therefore, Soviet authorities did not issue them any hard-currency travel allowance. This would prove to be very damaging to them when they were later arrested.

After her arrest, Lyalya spent a month in the terrible Sukhanovka prison, which was housed in a converted monastery. After a month, she began to cough up blood and was moved to Lubyanka prison. While a case against her was being built, she spent the next two years in Lubyanka prison sharing a cell with Alexandra ("Alya") Efron.[3] Incidentally, as a result of another one of those prison reshufflings, Alya Efron had spent the previous six months sharing a cell with Dynochka.

Both Alya and Dynochka survived their prison experience. They met again in Moscow in 1946, during a brief interval between Dynochka's arrests, and Alya described to Dynochka the last few months of her sister's life.

Lyalya's interrogator was Lavrenty Beria himself. He pressed her to name her own mother, Alexandra Kanel, and Polina Zhemchuzhina as spies. Returning to her cell after each interrogation, Lyalya complained that Beria was using hypnosis on her, because she found herself repeating everything he said and then signing her name to it.

When Dynochka's own case was nearing completion, she was given Lyalya's testimony to read. Lyalya had indeed admitted to everything they wanted... all of it: that her mother was a spy; that

---

[3] Alya Efron was the daughter of the great Russian poet, Marina Tsvetayeva. Although not directly related to these events, Alya's family also suffered a tragic fate. The family became separated in the turmoil of the Revolution and Alya's father, Sergey Efron, ended up in the West, where Marina Tsvetayeva and Alya eventually joined him. After Alya's brother Georgy ("Mur") was born, the family settled in Paris, living in poverty and alienation. The NKVD lured Efron and his family back to the Soviet Union where he and Alya were arrested in September 1939. Tsvetayeva and Mur remained free but destitute without any means of support as Tsvetayeva was denied employment. She hanged herself in 1941.

Polina Zhemchuzhina was a spy; that Lyalya herself had received money in Paris as payment for her mother's espionage activities, and that Dynochka knew about this...

In the 1950s, after Stalin's death and Dynochka's final release from prison, she and her husband Adolph received Lyalya's official death certificate stating that she had died of heart failure in January 1942. Like so many such notices, it was a sheer lie. Half a century later, Dynochka learned the truth about Lyalya's death. A document signed by Stalin, dated October 1941, was found in the archives. It was an instruction to deputy interior minister Bogdan Kabulov to have the death penalty carried out on a list of prisoners. Number five on the list was Yulia Veniaminovna Kanel (Lyalya). One hundred and sixty prisoners were executed by firing squad in a forest near the city of Oryol[4] in October 1941. Due to a fortuitous combination of events, Dynochka avoided the firing squad.

5. Dynochka and Her Miraculous Deliverance

At the time of her arrest, Dynochka was pregnant. She had had a miscarriage earlier and was excited to be expecting again. When she was told by prison authorities after her arrest that she had to have an abortion, Dynochka firmly refused. It is unclear why, having the power of life and death over their prisoners, the authorities troubled with such niceties as an inmate's consent, but they did and a stalemate ensued. Eventually, they placed a stooge in her cell, a young Komsomol woman who pestered her day and night telling her that prison was no place to have a baby and that

---

[4] Alya's father, Sergey Efron, was listed first in this execution list commissioned by Stalin. Numbers eleven and twelve were the widows of two top military commanders, Uborevich and Tukhachevsky; their husbands had been executed back in the 1930s.

she should have an abortion. The woman finally wore her down; Dynochka agreed and was taken from Lubyanka to the hospital at Butyrskaya prison. Butyrskaya had a much more lenient regime than Lubyanka. When an obstetrician arrived to perform the abortion and began preparing for the procedure, Dynochka noticed that there seemed to be no provision made for anesthesia. When she asked, the doctor confirmed that the procedure would be performed without anesthesia. Protesting vehemently, Dynochka withdrew her consent: "I won't let you do it without anesthesia!" The obstetrician — a doctor brought in from the outside, where such things still mattered — said to the prison doctor in attendance, "If the patient refuses, I will not perform the abortion." But the prison doctor sternly ordered him to begin, and so he did.

The pain was unbearable. Dynochka gave out heart-rending, agonizing screams. The obstetrician snapped, "Stop it! You are disturbing me. I can't work when you are screaming." But Dynochka went on screaming, right until the very end.

Afterward, she was taken to the Butyrskaya prison hospital ward, and five days later she returned to Lubyanka. A day after her return, she was summoned for an interrogation where she was beaten with a rubber club for refusing to "tell the truth" about her mother and Polina Zhemchuzhina being spies. A professional was brought in, a young man of about twenty, named Zubov. He beat Dynochka with his club for about five or ten minutes, until she could hold out no longer. She screamed, "Stop beating me! I'll say what you want." But the beating caused a massive uterine bleeding. She was in excruciating pain, unable to speak. The investigator sent her back to her cell where she fainted. By sheer coincidence, her cellmate at the time was Mischka whose extraordinary story had been described in the previous chapter. Mischka called for help. Dynochka was taken back to the Butyrskaya prison hospital and the same doctor who performed the abortion was called in to stop the bleeding — also without anesthesia, but this time Dynochka did not feel a thing because she was unconscious. She spent a week at the Butyrskaya hospital before being sent back to Lubyanka.

Miraculously, this ordeal — the abortion, the beating, and the subsequent bleeding — actually saved her life. During the week that she spent at the Butyrskaya hospital, important developments took place in the case against her. Her interrogations stopped.

Here is what happened. During that week, the Soviet Union signed the Molotov-Ribbentrop pact with Hitler. This major geopolitical event unexpectedly had an impact on one small life. Vyacheslav Molotov was appointed Foreign Minister and it was decided that his wife, Polina Zhemchuzhina, would not be arrested at that time (she would be arrested ten years later). Since she was no longer slated to be arrested, it was no longer necessary to beat confessions out of prisoners in order to implicate her in espionage. This saved Dynochka's life; she got away with "merely" two beatings and never had to implicate anyone, including herself. The charge of espionage against her was dropped and she was convicted of the comparatively trivial offense of failing to inform on the anti-Soviet activities of her relatives.

Dynochka was released from prison in 1953 after Stalin's death. A year later, Victor Abakumov, the former Minister of State Security (or MGB), was put on trial. Prior to his downfall, Abakumov had presided over an expansion of the MGB's authority, which came to include the full range of power to arrest, investigate, try, convict, and sentence individuals in Russia and Soviet-occupied nations, as well as to carry out death sentences. But at the end of 1951, Abakumov, denounced by his closest associate Mikhail Ryumin (the one who had instigated the Doctors' Plot), became a victim of Stalin's purges himself.

Abakumov's trial was actually intended to serve as the groundwork for a case against Lavrenty Beria, and once again Zhemchuzhina's case came up. The prosecutor, General Rudenko, revealed that in 1939, Beria had arrested twenty-five people in an attempt to obtain false testimony against Zhemchuzhina. Their names were read out in court and all but one had either been executed or died in prison: Yulia Kanel (Lyalya) was executed; her husband Severin Veinberg was executed; Zhemchuzhina's brother and sister died in prison; Zhemchuzhina's adopted sister was executed. The only survivor was Nadezhda Veniaminovna Kanel, or Dynochka, who was called to testify at the trial.

Also mentioned at Abakumov's trial was the second case against Zhemchuzhina, which had led to the arrest of a separate group of twenty-five people in 1949, again including Dynochka. By 1954, only four of them were still alive. They also gave testimony at the trial. Abakumov was sentenced to death and executed in December 1954.

One thing that all these victims had in common was their connection to the death of Stalin's wife, Nadezhda Alliluyeva. All in all, the lives snuffed out in the wake of her death number in the dozens, if not hundreds. The great Kremlin doctors, Dmitry Pletnyov and Lev Levin; Lyalya Kanel and her husband; Olga Kameneva and her sons; and many, many others... Stalin did not forget or forgive anyone he suspected of having knowledge of his crimes and cover-ups. Paradoxically, his major target, Polina Zhemchuzhina, survived the purges and died of natural causes.

These were the things Dynochka told me the night she came to see me after my father's funeral.

I was deeply shaken by her account. Was it really Stalin who said that the death of one person is a tragedy while the death of millions is a statistic? The scale of his carnage boggles the mind and makes the numbers seem somehow dry and abstract. Hearing Dynochka's first-hand account of her sufferings, and of the sufferings and deaths of her friends and family, made the sufferings and deaths of the dozens of millions of Stalin's victims become so much more real and horrible.

Life had a way of compensating some Gulag survivors for their lost years. Dynochka Kanel lived a very long life and passed away in Moscow only in the early 2000s, aged almost one hundred.

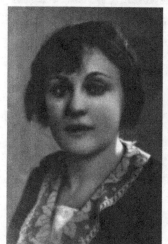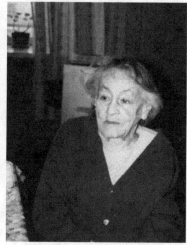

Dynochka Kanel in the 1930s (left) and in the 1990s (right).

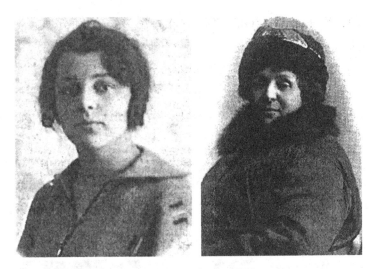

Lyalya Kanel (left) and Alexandra Kanel, the Head of the Kremlin Hospital in early 1930s.(right).

Chapter 9

The Mystery of Stalin's Wife's Death: Who Pulled the Trigger?

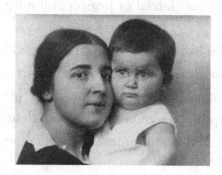

Nadezhda Alliluyeva with her daughter Svetlana (a photograph available in the public domain).

Dynochka Kanel's recollections presented in the previous chapter ignited my interest in Nadezhda Alliluyeva's death. I started my own research and collected information from various literary sources. My findings inspired me to reconstruct the events in the form of a mock trial of Joseph Stalin for the murder of his second wife.

The reader may recall that in the early morning of November 9, 1932, Nadezhda Alliluyeva, Stalin's second wife, was found dead in her room with a gunshot to her temple. The cause of her death was never officially disclosed, giving rise to a number of conflicting rumors. As Winston Churchill said, "A lie gets halfway around the world before the truth has a chance to get its pants on." Some rumors stated that Stalin shot her; others suggested that she shot herself in a fit of jealousy over Stalin's affair with a woman called Rosa Kaganovich. Stalin was clearly determined not to let the truth be known and viciously pursued everyone who was connected even the slightest with Nadezhda Alliluyeva's death.

We are left to wonder: was it suicide or was it murder? Although we may never know for sure, we can review the available information and separate fact from rumor. To that end, I propose to stage a mock trial of Joseph Stalin for the murder of his wife.

This won't be like one of those trials staged by Stalin where defendants are doomed even before being arrested — where they had no right to counsel, proceedings took only twenty minutes, no one was ever acquitted, sentences were pre-determined and not subject to appeal, and death sentences would often be carried out the same day.

Our trial will be infinitely fairer: a true adversarial proceeding with a prosecution and defense, each equally able to call witnesses and to give summations analyzing the credibility of conflicting witness accounts. I, the author, will be the judge, ensuring that each side gets its say. You, the reader, will be the jury; you will examine the evidence and make your decision.

Our single departure from the strict rules of procedure will be to admit hearsay testimony. No direct evidence of murder has ever been found; all existing accounts, even those of Nikita Khrushchev and Stalin's daughter, Svetlana Alliluyeva, are based on second- and third-hand information. At least different four groups of people gave varying accounts of the circumstances and cause of Alliluyeva's death. We will let them speak so we can reconstruct the most plausible scenario and decide whether it was Stalin himself who pulled the trigger of her small pistol.

Our trial opens with both sides presenting their opening statements.

1. Opening Statement: Prosecution

Your Honor, ladies and gentlemen of the jury. Joseph Stalin, the bloody Russian tyrant of the 20th century, needs no introduction. This is the man whose victims number in the millions; whose policies perfected and expanded a repressive regime where innocent people disappeared without a trace in the middle of the night into prisons and labor camps, imprisoned and tortured for crimes they didn't commit — to return as broken shadows of their former selves — or never to return at all.

Yet today our focus is on just one of these victims: Stalin's own wife, Nadezhda Alliluyeva, the mother of his two children, Svetlana and Vassily. We will hear testimony that shows that on November 8, 1932, Ms. Alliluyeva attended an exclusive dinner party with Stalin at the home of Marshal Kliment Voroshilov, a dinner for the top-ranking Party elite. We will hear that she left early after a quarrel with the defendant and was later found dead in their home, with a bullet wound in her temple. We will hear testimony that will establish that it was the defendant who pulled the trigger of the gun that killed her, and we will also hear what happened afterwards.

Today we will hear from *Nikita Khrushchev*. He, too, needs little introduction. Khrushchev is remembered today as the man who denounced Stalin's cult of personality after the dictator's death and succeeded him as head of the Soviet Union. But during the events in question he was just another unprincipled young man on the make, an eager accomplice in Stalin's purges. However, his testimony is important because he personally knew both the defendant and his wife: he had been her classmate at the Industrial Academy and was often invited to their home. This witness will tell us that the day before she died, Ms. Alliluyeva attended a parade where she seemed to be in good health and adequate mood.

Our next witness is *Nadezhda Kanel*. Her mother was the Head of the Kremlin Hospital who was pressured to sign a death certificate stating that Ms. Alliluyeva had died from appendicitis. Dr. Kanel refused to do so because she did not see the body and had been told by the Molotovs that the death had been from a gunshot.

Like so many innocent people caught in the wake of Ms. Alliluyeva's death, Ms. Kanel, the daughter, was arrested and spent time in Stalin's prisons. There, she was told — indeed, entrusted with — the story of Nina Uborevich, one of the guests at that fateful dinner party who related that Stalin had flirted with her at the party and then been terribly rude to his wife. Ms. Uborevich stated that she was later called to Stalin's home where she saw Ms. Alliluyeva's body on the floor with a bullet wound in her left temple, which is significant because Ms. Alliluyeva was right-handed.

Ms. Kanel also knew the pediatrician of Ms. Alliluyeva's children, Dr. Rosenthal, who was her mother's friend as well as a family friend to the deceased. Dr. Rosenthal told Ms. Kanel directly that the defendant had killed Ms. Alliluyeva.

Next, we will hear from *Aino Kuusinen*, a friend of another doctor, Dr. Muromtseva, who was called in to dress the body after it had been found. Dr. Muromtseva related another significant detail to our witness: the bruises on the victim's neck.

We will also hear from *Elizabeth Lermolo*, another victim of Stalin's repression and another one of those entrusted with eyewitness testimony while in prison. Ms. Lermolo's source was Natalia Trushina, a live-in housekeeper for the defendant and his wife. Ms. Trushina told our witness that the night after the party,

Stalin and his wife had a violent quarrel about his affair with a woman named Rosa Kaganovich, the sister of Stalin's close associate, Lazar Kaganovich, and they also quarreled about his leadership of the Party and his bloody purges and political murders. Ms. Trushina saw Stalin choking Ms. Alliluyeva with both hands; she screamed; Stalin broke away and ran out of the room, leaving Ms. Alliluyeva dead and blood-stained on the floor.

We will hear from *Dmitry Pruss*, a distant relative of Lazar Kaganovich, who will tell us that Rosa Kaganovich never existed.

Our last witness is *Yakov Dzhugashvili*, the son of Joseph Stalin and his first wife, Yekaterina Svanidze. Mr. Dzhugashvili, who was captured by the Nazis during WWII, will tell us that the rumors about Stalin's affair and marriage to Rosa Kaganovich had reached Germany and that his captors were very interested in her whereabouts, but that he decisively refuted her very existence.

Therefore, you will hear from witnesses that Ms. Alliluyeva was right-handed but was killed with a gunshot to her left temple. Also, Stalin was seen choking her and her neck showed finger marks. Finally, you will hear that Ms. Alliluyeva and Stalin had two quarrels that night. The first one caused her to walk out of the dinner party. The second was the one where Ms. Alliluyeva confronted him about his marital unfaithfulness as well as his murderous policies. That one turned violent, as our witnesses will tell us, and culminated in Ms. Alliluyeva's death.

Ladies and gentlemen of the jury, after hearing our evidence, we believe that you will agree with us that Joseph Stalin, the butcher of millions, has yet another life on his conscience: that of his young wife and mother of his children, Nadezhda Alliluyeva; we ask that you find the defendant guilty.

2. Opening Statement: Defense

Your Honor, ladies and gentlemen of the jury. We are not going to deny Joseph Stalin's reputation as a brutal and cold-blooded murderer of millions. These crimes are well-documented, but they are not what we are here today to examine. Today, we will show that, whatever else the defendant did, he did not personally murder his wife, Nadezhda Alliluyeva, on the night of November 8 or early morning of November 9, 1932.

We will hear from a member of Stalin's bodyguard who was on duty on the night of November 8, heard a gunshot coming from Ms. Alliluyeva's bedroom, and ran into the room to find her dead on the floor — alone.

We will also hear from Ms. Alliluyeva and Joseph Stalin's daughter, Svetlana, who was six at the time of her mother's death. Svetlana learned about the events of that night from her nanny, who told her that prior to Ms. Alliluyeva death, she had been deeply depressed and suffered from headaches. The nanny was the one who, together with their housekeeper, found the body on the floor of Ms. Alliluyeva's bedroom.

Svetlana also spoke with her mother's close friend, Polina Zhemchuzhina, who had witnessed the ugly scene between Stalin and his wife at the dinner party and accompanied her home from the party.

Importantly, Svetlana heard that Ms. Alliluyeva had left a letter addressed to Stalin, in which she expressed her deep disappointment with his leadership of the country.

We will also present two pieces of documentary evidence corroborating the existence and importance of Rosa Kaganovich, the sister of the defendant's close associate and member of the Politburo, Lazar Kaganovich. The first exhibit is an excerpt from

Stalin's obituary in the London Times, which states that after his wife's death, Stalin married Rosa Kaganovich. The second is an excerpt from a biography of Stalin written by the American historian, Robert Payne. Based on authentic documentary evidence, the book describes Ms. Alliluyeva's attendance at the parade on November 8 and notes that she looked pale and worn and took little interest in what was happening around her. It also recounts the quarrel at the dinner party and notes that it may have had to do with Rosa Kaganovich.

You will, therefore, be provided with evidence showing that Nadezhda Alliluyeva had suffered from depression, both over her disillusionment with her husband's political leadership and over his affair with Rosa Kaganovich. You will hear testimony showing that Ms. Alliluyeva was alone when she died. The combined weight of the evidence will establish that, whatever his other crimes, Joseph Stalin did not pull the trigger of the gun that killed his wife; she did it herself. After considering the evidence, we ask that you find the defendant not guilty.

***

3. Witness Testimony

The prosecution calls its first witness: Nikita Khrushchev.[1]

Prosecutor: *State your name for the record.*

NSK: Nikita Sergeyevich Khrushchev.

---

[1] Based on Khrushchev's memoirs, first published in the USSR in the 1970s and available in English from Penn State University Press: https://www.amazon.com/Memoirs-Nikita-Khrushchev-Commissar-1918-1945/dp/0271058536

P: *Did you personally know the deceased?*

NSK: Yes. She was my fellow student at the Industrial Academy. I was the leader of the Communist Party cell there and she was a member of the Communist Party committee.

P: *Were you friends with her?*

NSK: We were friends for a while. I believe she put in a good word for me to her husband, Comrade Stalin. It facilitated my rapid rise in the Party. But then Stalin ordered the purges of the "rightist" (Menshevik and Trotskyite) students and faculty at the Academy, and when I began carrying out the order, she became distraught because a number of her friends were among those arrested and who disappeared.

P: *Did you personally know the defendant?*

NSK: Yes. I knew him during these events and, of course, I came to know him better afterwards. In 1932, I began to be invited to participate in various meetings organized by Comrade Stalin, both formal and informal. We developed a good relationship. He liked to invite me to his dacha where we drank good Georgian wine and watched Western movies that were forbidden to the general viewer. We also discussed political problems. In March 1939, I became a full member of the Soviet Politburo.

P: *How did Stalin and his wife get along?*

NSK: I can only go by what I've heard. Sometimes, when Stalin was a little drunk, he would tell us things like: "I locked myself in my bedroom and she knocked on the door and screamed: 'You are an impossible man. It is impossible to live with you!' But I just kept the door locked and sat there while she kept calling me rude, callous, and inhuman…"

P: *Would you characterize the defendant as brutal and intolerant?*

NSK: Yes. Stalin amply demonstrated his intolerance, his brutality, and his abuse of power. Not only did he use repression and physical elimination against his actual enemies but also against people who had not committed any crimes. Everyone lived in fear in those days, expecting a fatal knock on the door in the middle of the night...

P: *What do you know about the cause of Nadezhda Alliluyeva's death?*

NSK: Well, of course, there was never a full official report. I and the other Party comrades just asked Nikolay Vlasik, the head of Stalin's bodyguards, what happened. He told us that after the October Revolution parade, everyone went to Voroshilov's place for dinner. That's what they did after parades: they always went to his place to eat; he had a big apartment. It was a very select group of people: the marshal of the parade, the members of the Politburo, and a few others. They went there straight from the Red Square. In those days, parades and demonstrations lasted a very long time, so everyone would eventually be hungry. Of course, there was a lot of drinking at dinner as usual. Vlasik said that Stalin came alone, without his wife, and left when everyone else did. I'm not sure of the exact hour, but it was very late. However, Stalin didn't go home apparently, and Nadezhda Sergeyevna became concerned. She put a call through to their dacha and asked the duty officer, "Is Stalin there?" "Yes," he answered, "Comrade Stalin is here." "Who is with him?" she asked. The officer gave her the woman's name... In the morning — I don't know exactly when — Stalin came home, and Nadezhda Sergeyevna was no longer alive. Vlasik said that the other woman was the wife of Sergey Gusev, one of the dinner guests. When Stalin left, he apparently took Gusev's wife with him and brought her to the dacha and slept with her, and that rookie fool, the duty officer, told Alliluyeva. She asked him and he just told her the truth.

P: *Do you consider Vlasik's account credible?*

NSK: Vlasik might have been misinformed; he was, after all, just a bodyguard.

P: *You have testified that you interacted with Ms. Alliluyeva at the Industrial Academy and were occasionally invited to her and the defendant's home. Did she strike you as a jealous woman?*

NSK: She didn't strike me as particularly jealous.

P: *Do you have different or additional information?*

NSK: The day before her death, during the parade in the Red Square, I stood next to Nadezhda Sergeyevna and we talked. She looked like a healthy, blooming young woman without any sign of depression. It was windy and Stalin stood on the Mausoleum with his overcoat unbuttoned. She looked up at him and said, "My man forgot his scarf again. He's going to catch a cold." The next day Kaganovich gathered the district Party secretaries and told us that Nadezhda Sergeyevna had passed away. I was shocked. She was a beautiful woman, very nice and hospitable, and we had talked just the day before. But of course, things happen, people die. However, two days later Kaganovich gathered us again and said, "Stalin has asked me to let you know that she did not simply die but had shot herself." Just like that! They never explained to us why she had done it. Later there were rumors that maybe Stalin had killed her. There were also rumors that Stalin had come into her bedroom with Voroshilov and found her dead. It is hard to say if that was true. After all, why would he bring Voroshilov along to go into his wife's bedroom? On the other hand, if he wanted to have a witness, it meant that he knew what he would find in there. Of course, if I heard these rumors, so did Stalin — he certainly knew about them from his agents. In a word, this part of the story is not clear.

P: *Do you know if Alliluyeva left a suicide note?*

NSK: She didn't leave a note; or if there was one, we never heard about it.

P: *Based on General Vlasik's account, Stalin spent the night after the party with the wife of Sergey Gusev. Did you ever meet Gusev or his wife?*

NSK: Vlasik said that Gusev was from the military, but I didn't know him, nor do I remember meeting his wife.

P: *Why weren't you at the party?*

NSK: I wasn't high up enough yet to be invited. Only the top brass were invited, like the commander of the parade — I think his name was Kork — and his commander, who was Voroshilov, and other people that were part of Stalin's closest circle.

P: *Were you acquainted with the high-ranked military officials of that time?*

NSK: I wasn't personally acquainted with every one of them, but of course I knew their names.

P: *But you had never heard of Gusev.*

NSK: That's right.

P: *Your honor, I have no more questions.*

Judge: *The defense may now question the witness.*

Defense counsel: *Stalin's daughter, Svetlana, wrote in her memoirs that Alliluyeva had left a suicide letter. You said that there was no letter. Are you sure that there was no letter and that Molotov or Voroshilov never mentioned it in connection with Ms. Alliluyeva's death?*

NSK: I'm not saying that there was no letter. I'm just saying that I never heard of one. It does not mean that there was no letter.

DC: *Thank you, no more questions.*

The prosecution calls the next witness: Nadezhda Veniaminovna Kanel.

P: *Please introduce yourself.*

Nadezhda Veniaminovna Kanel: I am Nadezhda Veniaminovna Kanel.

P: *Was your mother, Aleksandra Yulianovna Kanel, the Head Doctor of the Kremlin hospital at the time of Nadezhda Alliluyeva's death?*

NVK: Yes, she was.

P: *Did she tell you about Alliluyeva's death?*

NVK: Yes, when my mother came home from work on November 9, 1932, she told me and my sister Lyalya that Alliluyeva had committed suicide.

P: *Did she tell you that she had been requested to sign a death certificate?*

NVK: Yes, she told us that Stalin had wanted her to sign a certificate stating that Alliluyeva's death had resulted from appendicitis, but she refused to sign it because she had not seen the body. She had also heard from the Molotovs that Alliluyeva's death was from a gunshot wound.

P: *Did she tell you that other Kremlin doctors signed it?*

NVK: She told us that two of her colleagues, prominent Kremlin doctors Levin and Pletnyov, also refused to sign. But somehow news about the falsified certificate got out and circulated all over the country. Apparently, some other Kremlin doctor ended up signing it.

P: *Was an autopsy performed on Ms. Alliluyeva's body?*

NVK: No. On the evening of November 9, the casket with her body was transferred directly from her Kremlin apartment to the Grand Hall of the GUM building in Red Square, where the Government headquarters were then located. Public viewing opened early the next morning and continued until two hours before her funeral. She was buried at the Novodevichye cemetery on November 11 at 3 pm.

P: *Is your mother alive?*

NVK: No, she passed away.

P: *Did your mother die a natural death?*

NVK: My mother died suddenly and strangely. She had been a little sick for two days — a runny nose, a light fever, nothing serious; she was not bedridden. Then, unexpectedly, Yura Kamenev, the son of Lev Kamenev, arrived from Gorky. His father had been arrested. Yura was then 15 years old and he lived in Gorky with his mother who had been exiled there. He said that he needed to talk to my mother. They went into her study and stayed there for less than ten minutes. Yura came out and left right away. When my mother came out of the study, she looked terrible; her face had gone deathly pale with bright red spots. She did not tell us what was wrong. The next morning, we found her unconscious. She never regained consciousness and died two days later.

P: *Did the other two doctors who refused to certify Alliluyeva's death of appendicitis die from natural causes?*

NVK: No; Dr. Pletnyov and Dr. Levin were arrested and died in prison.

P: *Were you persecuted as well?*

NVK: Yes, my sister and I were also arrested. Our interrogators wanted us to sign statements saying that our mother was a spy and that Polina Zhemchuzhina, Molotov's wife and Nadezhda Alliluyeva's friend, was also a spy.

P: *And did you sign?*

NVK: No, I was lucky. They only beat me twice and I had enough strength left to will myself not to sign. I spent many years in prison, but I survived. My sister, however, did sign — and was executed.

P: *While in prison, did you meet any of the people who had attended the party at Voroshilov's apartment and witnessed the quarrel between Alliluyeva and Stalin?*

NVK: No, but I heard about it in 1949 while in prison at Novosibirsk from a Latvian woman named Austrin. She was my cellmate there. Ten years earlier, in Lubyanka prison, she had been a cellmate of Nina Uborevich, the widow of the top-ranked military commander, Jeronim Uborevich. When Uborevich and other prominent military commanders were arrested and executed in June, 1937, their wives were also arrested and kept in Lubyanka.[2] Nina Uborevich shared her story with Austrin in 1939 and asked her

---

[2] In 1941, after WWII had started and when the Germans were approaching Moscow, most Lubyanka prisoners were transferred to another prison in the city of Oryol, 220 miles south-west of Moscow. In October 1941, on Stalin's orders, one hundred and sixty prisoners (Nina Uborevich and other wives of executed military commanders among them) were taken to the Medvedev forest near Oryol and executed.

to remember it, write it down and preserve it after her release. Austrin's first prison sentence was supposed to be short, but when I met her ten years later, she was still incarcerated. Austrin shared Nina Uborevich's story with me.

P: *Did Marshal Uborevich and his wife attend the party at Voroshilov's apartment on November 8, 1932?*

NVK: Yes, Nina Uborevich and her husband were there. In fact, Nina did not merely witness the quarrel between Stalin and Alliluyeva; she was the cause of it. That evening, Stalin was drunk and very rude to Alliluyeva. He threw something at her — a piece of bread or a cherry pit — and then started flirting openly with Nina Uborevich. Nina tried to leave but Stalin caught her and ripped the veil off her hat. Alliluyeva became enraged with his behavior and left the party accompanied by her friend Polina Zhemchuzhina. They walked around the Kremlin for about forty minutes. Sometime after that, Stalin also left the dinner and went home. Austrin said that about twenty minutes after Stalin's departure, he phoned Nina Uborevich and asked her to come to his place right away, which she did. She saw Alliluyeva dead on the floor, with a bullet wound in her left temple. Alliluyeva was right-handed, so Uborevich concluded that Stalin had shot her. In accordance with Stalin's instructions, she lifted Alliluyeva off the floor, put her on the bed, tried to arrange her hair so as to cover the wound, and left.

P: *Ms. Kanel, has anyone else confirmed Ms. Uborevich's account as related by Ms. Austrin?*

NVK: Yes, but only the part about the dinner. After I was released from prison, I met Anna Rosenthal, a Kremlin pediatrician. She was the doctor of Alliluyeva's daughter Svetlana and a close friend of both my mother and Zhemchuzhina. Zhemchuzhina told her about her walk with Alliluyeva after they had left the party. During their walk, Alliluyeva complained bitterly about Stalin's appalling behavior. Zhemchuzhina tried to calm her down and then walked her home. As for the other part about Stalin calling Nina Uborevich and asking her to come and put his wife's body on the bed, I haven't met anyone who could confirm Austrin's story. I consider this to be prison folklore. But legends often carry a seed of truth, so Nina Uborevich's story could still be partially true. She certainly attended the viewing. Many people observed that Alliluyeva's head in the coffin was placed at a strange angle, presumably in order to conceal her wound. However, no one except Nina Uborevich appeared to notice that the wound was at Alliluyeva's left temple. As the wife of a military commander, Uborevich might indeed have noticed such details.

P: *Ms. Kanel, your mother's friend, Dr. Rosenthal, was Svetlana Alliluyeva's physician and a frequent visitor to Stalin's home. As Nadezhda Alliluyeva was always very busy, Svetlana was raised by her nanny. When the girl was sick, Dr. Rosenthal communicated more with her nanny than her mother. Dr. Rosenthal continued to provide medical care to Svetlana long after Alliluyeva's death. Surely, Dr. Rosenthal had knowledge about their family affairs. Did she tell you what she knew about the cause of Ms. Alliluyeva's death?*

NVK: Yes, Dr. Rosenthal told me that Stalin had killed Alliluyeva and that my mother knew that from Molotov and Zhemchuzhina.

P: *Your Honor, I have no more questions.*

Judge: *The defense may now question the witness.*

DC: *But surely, Ms. Kanel, Ms Austrin's account strains all credibility? For Stalin to ask Mrs. Uborevich for help in such a strictly private matter, she must have been his intimate friend. But was she? None of those who were close to the family ever mentioned Mrs. Uborevich as being part of Stalin's inner circle. Could you please comment on that?*

NVK: As I said, I believe that Austrin's story was at least partly a prison legend. I heard many such tales during my time in prison. Obviously, Stalin could not have phoned Nina Uborevich after he left the party, and her husband would never have let her go to Stalin's place alone. Was she secretly Stalin's lover? Surely not.

DC: *No more questions.*

The prosecution calls Aino Kuusinen.

P: *Please introduce yourself.*

AK: I am Aino Kuusinen, former wife of Otto Kuusinen, the founder of the Finnish Communist Party. He fled to the Soviet Union after the collapse of the 1918 Finnish revolution and eventually became a member of the Soviet Politburo. We married in the Soviet Union and divorced in 1930. Afterwards, I was posted to the United States and Japan while working for the Communist International, the Comintern. In 1938, I was arrested by the NKVD, imprisoned in Lubyanka, and spent fifteen years in prison and labor camps. In 1965, I managed to escape to the United States where I wrote and published my memoirs, entitled *Before and After Stalin.*

P: *Did you write in your book that Nadezhda Alliluyeva was murdered?*

AK: Yes.

P: *How did you know that?*

AK: On November 10, 1932, while I was in the United States, I saw the headline on the front page of the *New York Times* stating that Stalin had murdered his wife, Nadezhda Alliluyeva. My first reaction was that this could only be a malicious invention by the sensationalist bourgeois press. I did not believe it, but I also could not completely suppress my suspicions as references to the story kept cropping up in the press. The official Soviet version was that Stalin's wife had fallen seriously ill and died as the result of an operation; but what could have given rise to the rumor that she had been murdered?

I returned to Moscow at the end of the following July. The day after my arrival, I met with an old friend, Dr. Muromtseva of the Medical Academy. She was a loyal Communist who faithfully, and uncritically, defended all the strange things that were going on in the Soviet Union; her husband was a highly placed Old Bolshevik. After showering me with questions about life in America, which I answered to the best of my ability, she suddenly asked, "Did the American press say that Stalin murdered his wife?"

"Yes, the papers were full of stories about her death, and they did say she was murdered."

"And what did you think?"

"I didn't believe them."

"Well, it's true."

I stared at her in amazement and asked her how she knew, at which point she told me the following story.

"One morning, as I was just setting out for work, the telephone rang and an unknown man's voice told me to go straight to the guardroom at the entrance to the Kremlin and show them my Party card. Now, anyone in Moscow receiving such an order would be paralyzed with fear. I was no exception.

When I got to the Kremlin, the commandant was there with two other female doctors, and the three of us were taken down a hallway to Nadezhda Alliluyeva's room. She was lying on the bed, quite still, and we thought at first that she was ill and unconscious, but then we saw that she was dead. We were left alone in the room with the body of Stalin's wife. She had been a student at the Industrial Academy; her books and lecture notes were still on the table.

After a while, two men brought in a coffin and we were told by an official to place the body in it. We looked around for some appropriate clothing to dress her in and finally chose a black silk dress from one of the wardrobes. Suddenly, Dr. N. held up her hand to attract our attention and pointed to some black bruises on the corpse's neck. We looked closer and then exchanged silent glances — it was clear to all of us that she had been strangled. As we gazed at the body in horror, we saw the marks becoming larger and clearer until we could distinguish each finger of the murderer's left hand.

We then realized that when the body lay in state, anyone who saw the marks would know what the cause of death had been. Hence, we put a bandage around the neck so that the many thousands who came to pay their last respects to Nadezhda Alliluyeva would assume that she had died of some malady of the throat."

My friend ended her account with these words: "I'm sure you will understand when I say that the three of us have had many sleepless nights since then; we know too much."

Although the doctors thought that they had succeeded in hiding the truth, I found as I went around visiting old friends over the next few days that the rumor of Stalin's guilt was widespread. Most people thought he had attacked his wife in a fit of anger because she had confronted him about his policy of forced collectivization, which had brought misery and starvation to millions of peasants. The rumor was corroborated by the fact that after Alliluyeva's death, her relatives and other people who were connected with her, however slightly, began to disappear mysteriously.

It was, of course, extremely dangerous to breathe a word about the matter and it remained a taboo subject many years after. When I came back to Moscow in 1955 — twenty-three years after Alliluyeva's death and with fifteen years of prison and labor camps behind me — the murder was still a frequent topic of conversation.

Another friend of mine, also a longstanding Party member, told me a story she had heard from some of the Kremlin servants. Supposedly, Marshal Voroshilov, whose apartment was next to Stalin's, had heard Stalin's explosion of anger and Nadezhda's cries for help through his bedroom wall. He ran across in his night clothes to help her, but she was already dead.

P: *You honor, I have no more questions.*

Judge: *The defense may question the witness.*

DC: *Ms. Kuusinen, some of your statements require clarification. Here in my hands I have the November 10, 1932 issue of the* New York Times. *The newspaper did report on Alliluyeva's death on the front page. Here is the headline: "Stalin's Second Wife Dies Suddenly at 30; Cause Is Not Revealed, Accident Rumored." The article makes no mention of Stalin murdering his wife. Could you please comment on this?*

AK: I have no comments.

DC: *Secondly, Marshal Voroshilov's apartment in the Kremlin was not located next door to Stalin's. In fact, it was in a different building. Stalin lived in the Poteshny Palace while Voroshilov lived in the converted stables. Here is a plan of the Kremlin premises. The two buildings are clearly marked. There was simply no way Voroshilov could have heard Alliluyeva's cries for help, if in fact she had cried out. It was Molotov who lived in the same building with Stalin.*

AK: I simply described what I heard in Moscow from people I trusted.

DC: *Based on your report, Dr. Muromtseva and her colleagues found Ms. Alliluyeva lying on the bed in her bedroom. They dressed her in a black silk dress before placing her in the coffin. Had she been naked before that?*

AK: I have no comment.

DC: *Also, the three doctors were allegedly asked to put the body in the coffin. Is it common practice in the Soviet Union for medical doctors to place bodies in coffins before the authorities have a chance to examine the scene?*

AK: I have no comment.

DC: *Also, based on your report, Dr. Muromtseva described the marks on Ms. Alliluyeva's neck, which suggest that she had been strangled. She claimed that they could distinguish each finger of the murderer's left hand, which is clearly an attempt to incriminate the defendant, who — according to some rumors, which Dr. Muromtseva clearly believed — was left-handed; his right hand was said to be withered. But isn't it true, Ms. Kuusinen, that it was Stalin's left hand that was damaged in an accident in his youth, so he was actually right-handed?*

AK: I have no comment.

DC: *And finally, the marks on the deceased's neck simply could not have become larger and clearer several hours after death; that is a medical impossibility. Could you please comment on this?*

AK: I can only repeat what I have already said. I simply described what I heard in Moscow from people I trusted.

DC: *Thank you. Your Honor, I have no more questions.*

P: *You honor, may I pose another question to the witness?*

Judge: *Granted.*

P: *Ms. Kuusinen, you mentioned that the murder of Alliluyeva by Stalin was still a common topic of conversation for as long as twenty-three years after her death. In which circles did these rumors circulate? Among politicians?*

AK: Not necessarily. Due to Stalin's brutal and vicious personality, the general public readily accepted the assumption that he had murdered his wife.

P: *Thank you. Your Honor, I have no more questions.*

The prosecution calls Elizabeth Lermolo.

P: *Please introduce yourself.*

EL: I am Elizabeth Lermolo.

P: *Ms. Lermolo, did you serve time in Stalin's prisons?*

EL: Yes, I was arrested by the NKVD in 1934 after the assassination of Kirov and spent more than a decade in the islands of the notorious Gulag Archipelago. In 1950, I was lucky to escape from the Soviet Union to the United States. I wrote my memoirs and in 1955, my book titled *Face of a Victim* was published by the Harper and Brothers Publishing House. Among other things, I wrote what I knew about the death of Stalin's wife.

P: *What was the source of your knowledge? Did you meet somebody who witnessed her death?*

EL: Yes. In 1937, while I was incarcerated in the monastery prison in the old Russian town of Suzdal, I became ill and was taken to the prison hospital. My ward-mate in the hospital was a relatively young woman called Natalia Trushina. Although she was rather reserved, we eventually got to talking and she related to me her story.

Since her early youth, Natalia had lived with Nadezhda Alliluyeva's family for many years, first in Leningrad before moving with her to her Kremlin apartment in Moscow. Natalia was sort of a chaperone to Nadezhda. She was their housekeeper and stayed with the kids when Nadezhda was out. Because Natalia lived with the family, she knew many family secrets.

According to her, a new and strikingly beautiful woman suddenly appeared on the Kremlin stage. Her name was Rosa Kaganovich and she was a sister of Lazar Kaganovich, one of Stalin's leading henchmen and the only Jew on Stalin's leadership team. Rosa was a flamboyant brunette of about twenty-five, witty and sophisticated. Stalin was completely smitten. In the summer of 1932, he was a frequent visitor at Kaganovich's home in Silver Pines.

Nadezhda knew of this and the affair hurt her deeply. She knew that she could not win him back, so she concentrated on her studies and her upcoming graduation from the Industrial Academy. There was a strained atmosphere in their home during these months. Even Stalin's two children — Vassya (Vassily), who was then eleven, and Svetlana, who was nine — were aware of the new romance.

All the leading officials attended the November 8 party at Voroshilov's with their wives. Kaganovich came with his wife — and with Rosa — and Stalin came with Nadezhda. Natalia Trushina stayed home with the children. At about one o'clock that night, Alliluyeva returned home, escorted by Voroshilov, who left quickly. Nadezhda was hysterical: "They're going to kill me. That's my only future. I will be poisoned or killed in some sort of staged accident. Where can I go? What can I do?"

Natalia tried to calm her down. When she had quieted a bit, Natalia took her into the bathroom where, for no apparent reason,

Nadezhda fainted. Natalia did the first thing she could think of: she ran to the telephone, called Voroshilov's apartment and asked Stalin to return home at once. When he arrived a few minutes later, nervous and impatient, Natalia directed him to the bathroom. By this time Nadezhda had regained consciousness.

Through the partially opened door, Natalia heard the quarrel that followed. Nadezhda accused Stalin of carrying on shamelessly with "that woman" and of hurting and humiliating her. Stalin answered with a tirade. He told Nadezhda that she was no longer the right kind of companion for the leader of the world revolution, that his position put him above bourgeois concepts of morality, and that he needed someone to rekindle his spirit and revive his will to leadership. Nadya was infuriated. "Rosa revives you, I suppose!" And she went on, accusing him of usurping the Party's leadership by fraudulent means, of his bloody purges and liquidations, and of involving her in his shady schemes. "Shut up, damn you!" Stalin roared at last. Then Natalia heard a blow, a fall, someone gasping. Not quite knowing what she was up to, Natalia pushed open the door of the bathroom. There on the floor was Stalin, savagely choking Nadezhda with both hands. Natalia screamed, at which point Stalin broke away from Nadezhda and ran out of the bathroom. Nadezhda lay on the floor, not breathing. On her temple was a large wound that could have been from a blow with a blunt object. There was blood on her head, and near her on the floor was a bloodstained revolver.

Natalia carried her into the bedroom, bandaged the wound and put her ear to her heart but heard nothing. Then she rushed to the telephone to call a doctor, but at that moment, Stalin's secretary Poskrebyshev appeared and forbade Natalia to make the call. He went to the bathroom, hurriedly looked around, picked up the revolver, and ordered Natalia to clean up the bloodstains. A few minutes later, Voroshilov burst in, breathless, his eyes bulging. Without saying a word, he ran to see Stalin. After him came Molotov, sleepy, disheveled... Towards morning came Yenukidze, Nadezhda's godfather. He asked Natalia to help him with the corpse. Long before morning, Nadezhda's disfigured face was restored with the help of water, scissors, comb, cold cream and face powder, and her hair had been rearranged to conceal the wound.

The next morning, Natalia was taken to the monastery prison in Suzdal, with a promise that she would be released in a couple of weeks. She was still there in 1937.

P: *Ms. Lermolo, did you hear anything else about this woman, Rosa Kaganovich?*

EL: Yes. Later, when I was already in the West, I heard that the idea of Stalin's affair with Rosa Kaganovich originated in Paris in the late 1920s. It was floated by Russian-language press which was published, and read, by the exiled members of the White Guard who had fled from the Revolution and were anti-Communist and anti-Semitic in equal measure. The émigré press claimed that the Soviet Union was ruled by Jews through Stalin's mistress, Rosa Kaganovich. The émigrés feared that Lazar Kaganovich, a Jew, would become the next Russian leader and convert Russia into a "Jewish kingdom."

Stalin's death in 1953 gave rise to a new wave of rumors about Rosa Kaganovich, this time implicating her in Stalin's death. Some stories claimed that she had poisoned Stalin by order of Lazar Kaganovich in revenge for Stalin's persecution of Jews and his Doctors' Plot. Others, however, said that Rosa was seen, all dressed in black, sitting and sobbing next to Stalin's coffin.

P: *Your Honor, no more questions.*

Judge: *The defense may question the witness.*

DC: *Ms. Lermolo, I commend you on your very vivid description of the events of the tragic night of November 8, 1932. However, it raises some questions and I would like to hear your comments on them.*

In her book, Twenty Letters to a Friend, *Svetlana Alliluyeva mentioned their live-in housekeeper, an old German woman by the name of Karolina Til. She never mentioned Natalia Trushina as being a member of their household. Second, a person who had allegedly spent many years living in the family would have been expected to know the ages of Alliluyeva's two children, Vassily and Svetlana. Trushina said that Svetlana was nine at the time of her mother's death, but in fact she was only six. Moreover, you say that Natalia Trushina was arrested after Alliluyeva's death, but Svetlana's nanny was never arrested. How do you explain these discrepancies?*

EL: Well, my memory might have failed me on some points. I met Natalia Trushina in 1937 but I wrote my book fifteen years later, in the early 1950s. As to the name of the housekeeper, I have no comment.

The prosecution calls Dmitry Pruss.

P: *Please introduce yourself.*

DP: My name is Dmitry Pruss.

P: *What is your profession?*

DP: I am a geneticist by training.

P: *Are you related to the family of Lazar Kaganovich?*

DP: Yes, I am distantly related to them by marriage. More specifically, one of my ancestors married into the family. I have a keen interest in their family tree and have reconstructed it in detail. I know the dates and places of birth and death of nearly all of them, all the way back to the 19th century.

P: *Mr. Pruss, you have reconstructed the Kaganovich family tree. Does Rosa Kaganovich, the sister of Lazar, appear in that family tree?*

DP: No, sir. Lazar Kaganovich did have a sister, but her name was Rachel. She was a mother of four and died in 1926.

P: *Mr. Pruss, are you familiar with the name Stuart Kahan?*

DP: Yes. He was an American who came to Moscow from New York in 1987 and insisted on meeting with Lazar Kaganovich, who was still alive. Kahan claimed to be his grandnephew. Kaganovich vehemently denied the existence of such a relative, refused to meet with him, and even asked Andrey Gromyko, the Soviet Foreign Minister at that time, for help in protecting him from Kahan's advances.

This did not stop Kahan from publishing the book, *Wolf of the Kremlin: First Biography of L. M. Kaganovich, the Soviet Union's Architect of Fear*, upon his return to New York. It was released by William Morrow & Co in 1987. The book created a furor and has been widely cited. Amongst other things, Kahan detailed an alleged and long-lasting conspiracy against Stalin, according to which Kaganovich's sister Rosa had poisoned Stalin in 1953 with the consent of Molotov, Voroshilov, and others.

P: *Did Kahan identify the source of his information?*

DP: Yes, he claimed that the book was based on his conversations with Kaganovich during his visit to Moscow.

P: *Which, however, never happened?*

DP: Correct.

P: *No more questions.*

Judge: *The defense may question the witness.*

DC: *No questions for this witness.*

P: *Your Honor, the prosecution would like to read an exhibit into evidence. It is an excerpt from the rebuttal published by the family of Lazar Kaganovich against Stuart Kahan's book.*

Judge: *You may proceed.*

P: *Prosecution's Exhibit 1 reads as follows:*

"We insist that this book is filled with lies and slander. The author of the book falsely claims to be LMK's [*Lazar Moiseyevich Kaganovich — NR*] grandnephew in an attempt to persuade the readers to trust his writings. In fact, he is a fraud, and neither LMK himself, nor we ever had any idea about his existence. LMK vigorously denied the existence of any nephew in the USA. We…decisively refute these slanderous fabrications about LMK. The author claims that LMK supposedly introduced his sister into Stalin's household as a house doctor, and that several Politburo members, with her assistance, slowly poisoned Stalin. He also claims that this woman was "the dictator's wife." All this is a wicked calumny… The proof of the absurdity and falsity of this version lies in the fact that LMK's only sister, misnamed Rosa in the book (her name was Rachel), died in 1926 and was buried in Kiev at the Baykov Cemetery. She was married and raised five children. She never was a doctor, she never went to Arzamas, Nizhny Novgorod or Moscow, so she could not possibly have taken part in the actions the author insists on ascribing to her."

The prosecution calls Yakov Dzhugashvili.

P: *Please introduce yourself.*
YD: I am Yakov Dzhugashvili, the oldest son of Joseph Stalin and his first wife, my mother, Yekaterina Svanidze.

P: *What happened to your mother?*
YD: She died of typhus at the age of twenty-two, eight months after I was born.

P: *Was it your father who raised you?*

YD: No. I grew up in Tiflis (Tbilisi), Georgia, with my grand-mother, aunts, and uncle Alyosha. I was fourteen when I went to Moscow to live with my father, hoping eventually to go to university in Moscow. He was already married to Nadezhda Sergeyevna Alliluyeva, the deceased.

P: *You had had virtually no contact with your father until the age of fourteen. Did you get along with him once you started to live with him?*

YD: Oh, no, not at all! We had a very strained relationship. He despised me and took every opportunity to subject me to painful humiliation.

P: *Why do you think that was?*

YD: He looked down on me. To him, I was a provincial, a young oaf from the sticks. I knew little Russian when I came to Moscow and had to take lessons before I could get into university. I had no city manners. I was an embarrassment to him. Later, as I grew up and planned to marry, he took exception to both my choices. The first time I told him of my plans, the interview was so disastrously bad that my fiancée fled in tears, and I tried to kill myself. I failed; the bullet went through my lung but missed the heart. My father's only reaction was scorn: "You couldn't even do *that* properly." My second wife was Jewish, which infuriated him.

P: *Did you get along with your stepmother, Nadezhda Sergeyevna?*

YD: Oh, yes. She was very kind to me. She felt pity for me. I loved her and I think she loved me.

P: *Was it your father who sent you to the front when WWII broke out?*

YD: Yes, he said to me, "Go and fight." Unfortunately, I was captured by the Germans in mid-July, less than a month after the war started in the Soviet Union.

P: *Did the Germans know who you were?*

YD: Yes. I was interrogated by the Abwehr's best Russian experts. All my words were carefully written down.[3]

P: *What did they ask you?*

YD: Of course, first of all, they wanted to know about the condition of the Red Army and its war readiness. Then they asked about my father's family. Among other things, they were very interested in the whereabouts of someone called Rosa Kaganovich. They apparently believed that she was Lazar Kaganovich's sister and my father's third wife. I answered that I had never heard about this woman, her whereabouts, or her ties with my father.

P: *Was this true?*

YD: Absolutely. Even though I had a poor relationship with my father, if he had married again, I would have known about that from my relatives.

P: *Your Honor, no more questions.*

Judge: *The defense may question the witness.*

DC: *Mr. Dzhugashvili, was your father right-handed or left-handed?*

YD: He was right-handed. His left hand was damaged in an accident in his youth and was withered.

DC: *What year did your stepmother commit suicide?*

YD: I think it happened in 1934.

DC: *How old was your half-brother Vassily when it happened?*

YD: I cannot say exactly how old he was. Probably in his early teens.

---

[3] Based on information obtained from the Central Archives of the Russian Defense Ministry in Podolsk, as reported by various websites. The archives contain protocols of Yakov Dzhugashvili's interrogations by the Gestapo, which were seized by the English army and eventually passed on to the Soviet Defense Ministry.

DC: *Mr. Dzhugashvili, are you sure that your father was right-handed?*

YD: Yes. I know there was confusion about his damaged hand and there were rumors, but the man I grew up with was right-handed.

D: *Your Honor, no more questions.*

Judge: *Does the prosecution plan to call more witnesses?*

P: *No, Your Honor. The prosecution rests our case.*

Judge: *The defense may now call witnesses.*

The defense calls Nikolay Vlasik's subordinate, who was on duty the night of Alliluyeva's death.

DC: *Please tell us what your occupation was in November 1932.*

Guard: I was one of Comrade Stalin's bodyguards.

DC: *Were you on duty the night of November 8?*

Guard: Yes, my shift started at 10 pm.

DC: *Where was your post located?*

Guard: Outside the house, near Ms. Alliluyeva's bedroom window.

DC: *Did you hear a shot fired inside the house?*

Guard: Yes, I heard a shot coming from Ms. Alliluyeva's bedroom.

DC: *What did you do?*

Guard: I ran in there.

DC: *What did you see?*

Guard: She was lying on the floor in a black silk evening dress, her hair done up in curls. The pistol was on the floor.

DC: *Who else was in the room?*

Guard: No one. She was alone.

DC: *Your Honor, I have no more questions.*

Judge: *The prosecution may now question the witness.*

P: *What time was it when you heard the shot?*

Guard: I cannot say exactly. It was in the middle of the night. I was too shocked to look at my watch.

P: *What did you do next?*

Guard: I left her room and reported the incident to General Vlasik.

P: *What did he do?*

Guard: I don't know. I resumed my post outside the house. I was on guard duty.

P: *Are you sure that Ms. Alliluyeva was wearing an evening dress with her hair done?*

Guard: Yes, she was all dressed up.

P: *As if she had just come from a party?*

Guard: Yes, like that.

P: *Thank you, no more questions.*

The defense calls Svetlana Alliluyeva, daughter of Joseph Stalin and Nadezhda Alliluyeva.[4]

DC: *Ms. Alliluyeva, how old were you and your brother when your mother died?*

Svetlana Alliluyeva: I was six. My brother Vassily was eleven.

DC: *Do you remember your mother well? Can you tell us what she was like?*

---

[4] Based on Svetlana Alliluyeva's book *Twenty Letters to a Friend*, available in English from HarperCollins: https://www.amazon.com/Twenty-Letters-Friend-Svetlana-Alliluyeva/dp/0060100990

SA: She was very strict with us and never really petted us. She was more devoted to her husband than to her kids. It was Father who indulged us, or at least me, and I had real affection toward him. But despite being very busy and not paying much attention to us, Mother organized our education and leisure time very well. I had a great nanny and we also had excellent teachers. We grew up surrounded by many friends and had a happy childhood, up until her death.

DC: *Do you know the circumstances of your mother's death?*

SA: Well, for many years, I did not know anything about it. When I grew up and my Nanny became old and frail, she made a sort of confession to me, telling me about the events of the night of my mother's death. She told me that in the days before her death, Mother had been overtired, very sad and short-tempered, and had suffered from headaches and depression. My cousin later wrote that "there were people with weak psyches in our clan," ascribing my mother's suicide — if it was suicide — to the family's history of mental problems. My grandmother's sister, my great-aunt, was diagnosed with schizophrenia.

According to Nanny, several days before Mother's death, a classmate of hers came to visit. They sat and talked in our play-room, which Mother always used as her reception room. Nanny overheard some of their conversation. Mother kept saying that she was sick and tired of everything and nothing made her happy anymore. The friend asked, "Not even your kids?" Mother answered, "Nothing at all. Not even the kids." It sounded like she did not want to live any more. But, of course, no one could imagine that in two days she would be dead.

On the night of November 8, at the party in Voroshilov's apartment, Father was very rude to her. He shouted at her, "Hey, you! Drink!" She responded, "Don't you 'Hey you' me!" and left the party.

DC: *Do you know if your mother ever considered divorcing your father?*

SA: Yes, both our relatives and her friends later told me that she had often thought about divorce. But she was a person of duty, first and foremost; she took her obligations to her husband, her home and her children far too seriously. So, I don't think she would have ever left my father, even if she had occasionally considered it.

DC: *When and how was the body of your mother found?*

SA: My parents had separate bedrooms. Father's bedroom was to the left of the dining room. Mother's bedroom was to the right of the dining room, at the end of the same hallway that our bedrooms were on, a long way away from the service rooms. The windows of her bedroom looked out into the Aleksandrovsky garden.

According to Nanny, our housekeeper, Karolina Vassilievna Til, a nice old lady of German origin, used to wake Mother up in the morning. On the morning of November 9, as usual, Karolina Vassilievna cooked breakfast in the kitchen and went to wake her up. Then, trembling all over, she ran to our bedroom to get my Nanny. She could not speak. Karolina and Nanny ran to Mother's bedroom together. She lay on the floor near her bed, covered in blood. She was already cold. Beside her was a small Walther pistol that her brother Pavel, my uncle, brought over from Germany and gave to her. It wasn't loud enough to be heard in the service rooms.

Terrified that Father might come in at any moment, Nanny and Karolina lifted her, put her on the bed and cleaned her up. Then, not knowing what to do next, they ran to call people they considered the most important: Mother's closest friend, Polina Zhemchuzhina, and the chief of the guards. Soon everyone came running. They were shocked and could not believe their eyes. Father was still asleep in his bedroom. Finally, he came out into the dining room. They told him, "Joseph, Nadya is no longer with us."

DC: *Do you consider your nanny's account fully credible?*

SA: I believed it because my Nanny was a simple woman and would hardly have made it up.

DC: *Did anyone else confirm your nanny's account?*

SA: As far as their quarrel at the dinner party goes, yes. When Mother's friend, Polina Zhemchuzhina, returned from exile in 1953, she gave me a detailed account of the events that had taken place at Voroshilov's apartment on November 8, 1932. Zhemchuzhina had been there with Molotov and others. Everyone witnessed the quarrel between my parents, but no one thought much of it because my parents quarreled all the time. They disagreed on many things, including Father's Georgian habit of giving us and other kids Georgian wine. Mother did not like drinking — wine made her sick — and she did not like it when other people drank, either. It may have been a premonition: my brother Vassily later died of alcoholism at the age of forty... Zhemchuzhina told me: "Nadya was very angry with Stalin over his behavior at the party and left early. I went with her because I did not want to leave her alone."

DC: *Did you hear about the suicide letter that your mother left for your father?*

SA: I was told later that Mother left a letter addressed to Father. It was filled with accusations and reproaches. It was not just a personal letter; it was kind of a political letter, and it was a horrible letter. Mother had come to realize that Father was not the man she had thought he was, and she was incredibly disappointed.

Father was beside himself with rage. The letter was destroyed and I never saw it. I was told that he appeared shocked and bewildered by Mother's death. He felt that she had stabbed him in the back.

He was so shocked that during the viewing of the body at the civil farewell ceremony, when he came up to the coffin, he suddenly pushed the coffin away, turned around and left. He did not attend the funeral. In the normal course of events, Mother's body would have been cremated and her ashes placed in the Kremlin wall. For some reason, he gave orders that she be buried at the ancient aristocratic cemetery of the Novodevichy monastery. He never visited her grave.

DC: *Your Honor, I have no more questions.*

Judge: *The witness may now be questioned by the prosecution.*

P: *Ms. Alliluyeva, you have stated that your grandmother's sister was diagnosed with schizophrenia. Was your grandmother diagnosed with a mental illness?*

SA: No.

P: *Was your grandfather, your mother's father, diagnosed with a mental illness?*

SA: No.

P: *What about your mother?*

SA: No.

P: *When you were children, did your brother tell you that your father was Georgian and that Georgians were people who dressed in long coats known as the Chokha (in Russian, "cherkeska") and went around stabbing everyone with their daggers?*

DC: *Objection! Irrelevant!*

Judge: *Sustained.*

DC: *Your Honor, the defense would like to read two exhibits into evidence. Exhibit 1 is an excerpt from an obituary of Joseph Stalin which was published by the* London Times *between March 6 and 7, 1953.*[5] *Exhibit 2 is an excerpt from a book by Robert Payne,* The Rise and Fall of Stalin (Simon & Shuster, New York, 1965). *Both exhibits authenticate the existence and role of Rosa Kaganovich in Nadezhda Alliluyeva's death.*

Judge: *You may proceed.*

DC: *Exhibit 1 reads as follows:*

"Only a few-details are known of Stalin's personal life. In 1903 he married Yekaterina Svanidze, a profoundly religious woman and the sister of a Georgian comrade, who left him a son Yasha when she died in 1907 of pneumonia. His second wife, whom he married in 1918 — Nadezhda Alliluyeva — was 20 years younger than himself and was the daughter of a Bolshevik worker, with whom Stalin had contacts in both the Caucasus and St. Petersburg. She was formerly one of Lenin's secretaries and later studied at a technical college in Moscow. This marriage, too, ended with the death of his wife in November, 1932. She left him two children — a daughter, Svetlana, and a son, Vassili, now a high ranking officer in the Soviet Air Force. Late in life he married Rosa Kaganovich, the sister of Lazar Kaganovich; a member of the Politburo."

Exhibit 2 reads as follows:

"On November 7, 1932, the fifteenth anniversary of the Revolution was celebrated with a military parade on the Red Square. This

---

[5] Cited by http://www.thetimes.co.uk/tto/viewArticle.arc?articleId=ARCHIVE-The_Times-19 53-03-06-07-001&pageId=ARCHIVE-The_Times-1953-03-06-07

was followed by processions of workmen and athletes. As usual Stalin took the salute from Lenin's mausoleum. Nadezhda was seen among the crowds watching the display of military power. She looked pale and worn, took little interest in what was happening around her, and hung on her brother's arm. In three weeks she would receive her diploma as a chemical engineer, and her nervousness was perhaps no more than the inevitable nervousness of a woman who will soon leave the familiar surroundings of a college. She did not yet know what she would do with the knowledge she had acquired, but there were innumerable factories and laboratories in the Moscow region where her services would be welcomed. She could become an engineer working for the Soviet Union without leaving her family in the Kremlin.

Among the Soviet hierarchy the anniversaries of the Revolution were celebrated like Christmas. All-night parties continued sometimes through the day and the following night; innumerable toasts were drunk; presents were exchanged; there was a constant round of visits.

On the night of November 8 Stalin attended a party given at the country house of Voroshilov. He was accompanied by Nadezhda, and a small circle of intimate friends now reduced by the butcheries of the previous twelve months. At such parties he was always inclined to drink dangerously. Something said by Nadezhda — it may have been about another woman, Rosa Kaganovich, *who was also present*, or about the expropriations in the villages which doomed the peasants to famine — reduced Stalin to a state of imbecile rage. In front of her friends he poured out a torrent of abuse and obscenity. He was a master of the art of cursing, with an astonishing range of vile phrases and that peculiarly obscene form of speaking which the Russians call matershchina. Nadezhda could stand it no more, rushed out of the room, drove to the Kremlin and went straight to the small house where she had spent most of her married life. She died about four o'clock in the morning.

The official communique announced only that her death was 'sudden and premature.' No further official announcement was made, although a semiofficial report that she had died of acute appendicitis was circulated. Since she was not in good health and had looked wan and exhausted during the last months, it was generally accepted that the official report was true or alternatively that she had taken an overdose of sleeping pills. There were also rumors that she had shot herself through the head… She was thirty years old. In her short life she had little impact on the Russian scene."

DC: *Your Honor, I have no more witnesses. The defense rests.*

Judge: As no more witnesses have been called, we will now proceed to closing statements.

4. Closing Statement: Prosecution

Your Honor, ladies and gentlemen of the jury. I will now compare and analyze the information we collected during the trial.

Let me start by going over the facts that are not in dispute. Unfortunately, they are few. We know that on October 8, 1932, Nadezhda Alliluyeva marched in a parade celebrating the 15th Anniversary of the October Revolution. Later that night, she and Joseph Stalin attended a dinner party at Marshal Kliment Voroshilov's apartment in the Kremlin, where they quarreled — but no one thought much of it because they quarreled all the time. We also know that she left the party before Stalin did and that she walked around the Kremlin grounds for about forty minutes with her friend Polina Zhemchuzhina. The last thing we know for sure is that in the early morning of November 9, Alliluyeva was found dead with a bullet wound in her temple. Our knowledge of the established facts ends here.

Let us now consider the defendant's personality as we know it today. The defendant is a blood-thirsty tyrant responsible for the deaths of many millions of people. He was already starting down this violent path during his wife's lifetime. He was enjoying his omnipotence and his impunity, and he was starting to kill innocent people — ordinary people selected at random — in mass numbers. He organized murders of his political rivals or those whom he considered his rivals. Then he killed his rivals' killers. He used the murders as an excuse to get rid of other members of the opposition by accusing them of killing his rivals and then ruthlessly killing them for it. He killed anyone he suspected of supporting him less than wholeheartedly.

Ladies and gentlemen, you heard Stalin's own daughter Svetlana testify that the victim, Nadezhda Alliluyeva, did not fully approve of her husband's policies of fear and atrocities. Ask yourselves: how would a man of his character, who demanded absolute, unthinking loyalty — both personal and political — feel about this? Wouldn't he view it as an ultimate betrayal? And if so, it's not hard to see him taking action to stamp it out — by killing her.

Let us now consider the testimony of Ms. Lermolo. Of course, like most other witnesses we heard from today, Ms. Lermolo recounted events that have receded far into the past; hence some of her testimony must be discounted. Some, but not all. I invited Ms. Lermolo here to draw your attention to one particular aspect of her testimony. Ms. Lermolo testified that on the night of his wife's death, Stalin remained cool when Alliluyeva accused him of adultery but lost his temper and killed her in a fit of rage once she started criticizing his policies and his purges and murders. This is quite perceptive — and it is consistent with the testimony of the daughter of Stalin and Nadezhda, Svetlana.

You will recall that Svetlana testified that her mother left a letter addressed to her father that was, at least in part, an attack on his leadership. We can now surmise that Alliluyeva wrote this letter upon her return home after the quarrel at the party. Svetlana was told that it was not just a private letter but a "horrible" political letter showing that, during the last years of their life together, Alliluyeva's views had evolved toward those of Stalin's opposition — a fact which until then, we may assume, he was unaware.

While the defense has called this letter a suicide note, let us note that it is extremely rare for suicidal people to write political letters. There are, however, things that are much easier to express in writing than orally — the writer may be assured of getting her point across uninterrupted, and the recipient cannot turn his back and lock himself in a different room.

We may now attempt to reconstruct the events of that night. Let us assume that Alliluyeva either gave the letter to Stalin upon his return or left it in his room. When he returned home from the party, he read the letter and realized that his wife no longer gave his policies her unquestioning support but was now leaning toward his opposition in her views. Shocked and enraged, Stalin ran to her bedroom. A heated argument followed and, in a fit of rage, he grabbed her pistol and killed her. He was smart enough not to destroy her letter but to leave it in her room until morning to make it look like a suicide. Svetlana did not say who it was that found the letter, but it would certainly be one or more of those who had rushed to Stalin's home after the news: Polina Zhemchuzhina, the Head of the Guards, Kliment Voroshilov and Vyacheslav Molotov. The letter was destroyed at some point, but by then it had been read and it had done its work: the letter deeply wounded Stalin. Even Alliluyeva's death did not cool his rage — he pushed her coffin away at the viewing and did not attend her funeral.

The defense will have us believe that Nadezhda Alliluyeva's death was a suicide, but none of the alternative explanations presented to us have any merit. Let us begin with the testimony of Svetlana Alliluyeva's nanny. The nanny told Svetlana that in the early morning of November 9, she and the housekeeper, Ms. Til, found Nadezhda Alliluyeva's body near her bed, already cold and "all covered in blood." So what did they do? They called Zhemchuzhina and the Head of the Guards. Why didn't they call Stalin, who allegedly slept just a couple of doors away from the room? Wouldn't that have been the first thing to come to mind? Or did they have reason to know that Stalin was not asleep? Why then were the nanny and Ms. Til so afraid that he would enter the room? These are discrepancies that cast doubt on the nanny's testimony. They should make you question whether the nanny told Svetlana the whole truth about her mother's death.

Besides, even a simple, uneducated peasant woman like Svetlana's nanny should have known not to touch or move a blood-covered body lying on the floor with a pistol next to it. Yet, the nanny claimed that she and Ms. Til lifted Nadezhda, put her on the bed, and only then called for help. This, too, is not believable.

Let us now compare the nanny's story with that of Dr. Anna Rosenthal, as told to Ms. Kanel. Dr. Rosenthal was Svetlana Alliluyeva's pediatrician. Svetlana testified that her mother was always busy and never gave much time to her children. Little Svetlana grew up with her nanny, who was her best friend. We may conclude from this that when Svetlana was sick and Dr. Rosenthal was called in to attend her, she would speak with Svetlana's nanny rather than her mother.

As you may recall, Dr. Rosenthal told Ms. Kanel that Stalin had killed Alliluyeva and that Ms. Kanel's mother, the Head of the Kremlin hospital, knew about it. How could Dr. Rosenthal know that Stalin killed Alliluyeva? Who was her source of information? There are two possibilities: it was either Svetlana's nanny or Polina Zhemchuzhina, the victim's closest friend and the last person — except perhaps Stalin himself — to see her alive. Doctor Rosenthal was on friendly terms with Zhemchuzhina, but the nanny said that she and Ms. Til called Zhemchuzhina *after* the victim's body had been found. Therefore, Zhemchuzhina could not have been the primary source of information on the cause of Alliluyeva's death. The most reasonable conclusion is that it was Svetlana's nanny who told both Rosenthal and Zhemchuzhina that Stalin killed his wife.

Why then did the nanny not tell Svetlana this when Svetlana grew up? I think Svetlana's familial affection toward her father provides enough of an explanation. Svetlana loved her father despite what she knew about his actions. Her memoirs show a daughter's natural desire to see him as gentle and humane. In particular, she blames the monstrous deeds and atrocities of Stalin's era on his chief of secret police, Lavrenty Beria. Knowing this, we can reasonably assume that the nanny would wish to spare Svetlana, who was troubled enough by the knowledge that her father had murdered millions of people, including her own relatives and close friends. The three women — the nanny, Anna Rosenthal, and Zhemchuzhina — may well have made an agreement to keep the secret of Alliluyeva's death from Svetlana so long as they lived.

Do we have other evidence to confirm the murder theory?

Yes, indeed. You will recall the story of Ms. Nina Uborevich as related by Ms. Austrin to Ms. Kanel. Now, I will admit that as many as ten years had passed between Uborevich relating her story to Austrin and Austrin relating it to Ms. Kanel, and some of the details might have become garbled in transmission, but we have no evidence of any intentional distortion. I will even agree that the part where Ms. Uborevich found the body and lifted it off the floor and onto the bed is the least plausible part of the story. There are, in fact, no fewer than three people claiming to have lifted the body off the floor: Ms. Uborevich, the nanny, and Natalia Trushina. But even so, one part of Uborevich's story deserves our serious consideration — her statement that Alliluyeva's wound was at her *left* temple. Whether or not Uborevich was present at the scene immediately after the death, she certainly saw the victim later at the viewing and at the funeral. As the wife of a military commander, she would have noticed the placement of the wound and would have thought it significant, given that the victim was known to be right-handed. The position of the wound at the left temple of a right-handed person is strong evidence against self-inflicted death and supports the theory of murder. Unfortunately, as Ms. Kanel testified, no autopsy (which could have supported or disproved Ms. Uborevich's story) was ever performed on the body.

Let us now consider the story of General Vlasik, the head of Stalin's bodyguards, as related to us by Nikita Khrushchev. We can safely assume that General Vlasik's story is a fabrication: there are too many details that don't match any of the other stories. First, General Vlasik claimed that Stalin attended the party without his wife, when all surviving guests assert that they came together. Moreover, the guard who was on duty that night testified that he found Ms. Alliluyeva on the floor dressed in a black silk evening dress, with her hair done up in curls. She wouldn't dress up like that for a quiet evening at home, would she?

Second, only the highest-ranking military officials and Party leaders were invited to the party. General Vlasik claimed that one of the guests was Sergey Gusev, whose wife Stalin allegedly spent the night with at his dacha. To have been invited to that elite event, Gusev must have held a position or rank of some prominence; yet Nikita Khrushchev, already a member of Stalin's inner circle at that time, had never heard his name.

Third, other surviving guests have stated that Stalin left the party soon after Alliluyeva's departure and walked straight home to his Kremlin apartment. No one else has talked about a tryst at the dacha except for Nikolay Vlasik.

Why, then, give any attention to his story? We assert, ladies and gentlemen, that General Vlasik's story is important, not for what it says, but because it exists at all. Vlasik lied to Nikita Khrushchev and other Communist Party officials. He was clearly trying to create an alibi for the defendant, meaning that he was aware that his boss would need an alibi. Vlasik's story is part of a cover-up designed to present Alliluyeva's death as a suicide due to jealousy, to conceal the true cause of death: murder by Stalin.

You will recall that the theory of suicide due to jealousy is at the core of the entire case for the defense, although the object of Nadezhda Alliluyeva's presumed jealous fit is different: this time, it's not the wife of Sergey Gusev but a woman called Rosa Kaganovich, a sister of Lazar Kaganovich, one of Stalin's closest henchmen and the only Jew in his inner circle. Yet, as the evidence shows, this theory is the product of the purest fancy.

In fact, as Ms. Lermolo has testified, the idea of Stalin's affair with a Jewish woman originated in Paris in the late 1920s, during Alliluyeva's lifetime. It was floated in the Russian-language press published, and read, by the exiled members of the White Guard who had fled from the Revolution and were equally anti-Communist and anti-Semitic. The émigré press claimed that the Soviet Union was ruled by Jews through Stalin's mistress, Rosa. The émigrés feared that Lazar Kaganovich, a Jew, might become the next Russian leader who would convert Russia into a "Jewish kingdom."

The story of Rosa Kaganovich spread across Europe. You have heard it advanced by reputable sources, like Stalin's obituary in the *New York Times* or the American historian Robert Payne. You have also heard it put forth by another American author, Stuart Kahan, who claimed to be a great-nephew of Lazar Kaganovich and to have met with Kaganovich during his visit to Moscow in 1987.

However — and most importantly — Lazar Kaganovich himself firmly denied Rosa's existence throughout his long life, as did his family. You have heard from Dmitry Pruss, who read to us a rebuttal of Stuart Kahan's story that was published by the Kaganovich family. According to them, Lazar Kaganovich did have a sister, but she was not named Rosa and she was an older woman who would have been closer to fifty at the time of Alliluyeva's death — not the fiery younger beauty of the legend. She was a married woman with four children who never lived in Moscow, and most importantly, she died in 1926, six years before Alliluyeva's death.

Similarly, Stalin's own son, Yakov — who presumably would know of something as major as his father's remarriage — also denied Rosa's existence when captured by the Nazis.

Ladies and gentlemen, now that you have heard the evidence, I submit to you that the story of Rosa Kaganovich is a myth. Nadezhda Alliluyeva did not kill herself in a fit of jealousy over Stalin's dalliance, be it with Rosa Kaganovich or Mrs. Gusev.

The defense has also introduced evidence that Ms. Alliluyeva was suffering from depression in the final days of her life. Svetlana's cousin told her that her great-aunt was diagnosed with schizophrenia. Now that we have refuted the possibility of suicide from jealousy, let us consider suicide from mental illness. I believe that this version has no more merit than the first. It is true that mental illness tends to run in families, but the only documented case of mental illness we know of in Ms. Alliluyeva's line is her great-aunt, her grandmother's sister — a fairly distant relation. Neither of her parents were diagnosed with mental illnesses.

The circumstances of Ms. Alliluyeva's life offer ample reasons for the kind of symptoms she displayed. Consider that she was two weeks away from defending her thesis, a culmination of her entire school career. Who doesn't suffer from headaches on the lead up to a major, stressful event like that? Second, consider the suicide letter which, as Svetlana has testified, was not of a merely personal nature but had leveled political accusations at her husband. Here was a woman who had become disillusioned with her husband and the father of her children, the man she had once loved and even idolized. This man arrested and imprisoned her school friends, thus isolating her. This man had embarked upon the bloody career of a callous murderer, a criminal, and she had come to realize this. She was disillusioned in him as a man and as the leader of the country. No, ladies and gentlemen, we don't need to go around looking for hypothetical mental illnesses. These facts, right here, are sufficient to produce symptoms of depression in an otherwise healthy woman.

A woman, moreover, who was not without options. As we have said, Nadezhda Alliluyeva was two weeks away from receiving her chemical engineering diploma, which offered her the possibility of a professional career, of independence. Her future lay before her. There was nothing to prevent her from getting a job and, if she so chose, leaving Stalin, moving out and beginning an independent life. Although her daughter, Svetlana, believes that her mother's sense of duty would have prevented her from leaving, isn't suicide a much more grave — and more final — dereliction of that duty?

No, ladies and gentlemen, we have heard no credible evidence to support the theory of suicide. Nadezhda Alliluyeva did not kill herself either from jealousy or from depression.

There are, however, strong reasons to believe that Stalin personally murdered his wife, and that the murder was triggered by her letter condemning his way of ruling the country, his hypocrisy, and his murders and other crimes. Stalin killed her in a fit of rage after realizing that she had come to espouse the views of the opposition. That was his motive. There is also his character to consider based on his other actions. Let us not forget that he did kill many members of her family, his political opponents, real or imaginary, and many millions of innocent people.

I ask that you find the defendant guilty.

5. Closing Statement: Defense

Your Honor, ladies and gentlemen of the jury. Once again, we do not deny Joseph Stalin's history as a mass murderer. But the facts of each crime must be established independently. Although the prosecution wants you to believe that he killed his wife because he was a killer, the prosecution bears the burden of proving its case; and this the prosecution has failed to do.

None of the evidence presented by the prosecution is credible. I want to start with the testimony of Elisabeth Lermolo. Ms. Lermolo, who also wrote a book about these events, has undeniable literary talent, a gift of invention and misrepresentation. For example, consider the story of Natalia Trushina, the only person among all those we heard of today who had allegedly witnessed Stalin killing his wife. How likely is it that an eyewitness to such a murder would still be alive, five years later, to tell her story to Ms. Lermolo — especially when others with much more distant ties to Ms. Alliluyeva were killed for those ties?

In fact, who was Natalia Trushina — did she even exist? This woman supposedly lived in Alliluyeva's home for at least thirteen years as her companion and housekeeper, yet she did not know the age of her daughter at the time of Alliluyeva's death. Moreover, Svetlana Alliluyeva has testified that their housekeeper was an old German woman by the name of Karolina Til; no one we heard from today, aside from Ms. Lermolo, has mentioned Natalia Trushina. These inconsistencies are serious enough to cast substantial doubt on Ms. Lermolo's description of Stalin murdering his wife.

No more believable is the testimony by Ms. Aino Kuusinen, who would have us believe — citing Dr. Muromtseva — that three doctors saw finger marks on the victim's neck and could tell that these marks had been left by someone's left hand. There are so many things wrong with this story, one hardly knows where to start. First of all, one hand, ladies and gentlemen! I don't know about you, but I do believe that a murderer would normally try to use both hands, unless he was unusually strong and had unusually large hands — and the defendant was not a large man. The left hand itself presents a second problem. Ms. Kuusinen — or was it Dr. Muromtseva? — apparently believed rumors that the defendant was left-handed and used them to try to implicate him. In fact, ladies and gentlemen of the jury, Stalin was right-handed; it was his left hand that was injured in an accident in his youth. This has been confirmed for us by his own son, Yakov Dzhugashvili, who would surely know such a personal detail about his own father. And finally, Ms. Kuusinen would have us believe that those finger marks changed their appearance before the doctors' very eyes, several hours after the death, becoming larger and more distinct — which is simply medically impossible.

The testimony of Ms. Uborevich, recorded decades after it was related, likewise defies belief. To begin with, why was she even on the scene? This was a family tragedy, a strictly private matter. One would think that the family would want it contained as much as possible and not involve outsiders. Yet we are asked to believe that not only did Stalin ask Ms. Uborevich to come but he even asked her to lift his dead wife's body from the floor. What does this tell us about Ms. Uborevich? That she would have had to be one of the closest insiders, perhaps even an intimate friend of his. But none of the others who were close to the family ever mentioned Ms. Uborevich as being part of Stalin's inner circle.

And then, of course, the central fact on which the prosecution's theory of murder depends — the placement of the fatal wound on Nadezhda Alliluyeva's temple — is very much in question. The prosecution has made much of the fact that the wound was located on her left temple despite the victim being right-handed. Yet, as we have just discussed, neither of the two pieces of testimony placing it there — Ms. Kuusinen's and Ms. Uborevich's — are remotely believable. If that is the foundation of the prosecution's case, the case for murder must fail.

Finally, what about that suicide letter that Nadezhda Alliluyeva supposedly wrote to Stalin? We have heard from no one who read or even saw the letter. We don't know what it said. Everything about the letter is pure conjecture and cannot support the theory of murder.

Ladies and gentlemen, no *credible* testimony presented here contradicts the hypothesis that Nadezhda Alliluyeva committed suicide in a fit of jealousy toward Rosa Kaganovich.

The existence of Rosa Kaganovich that the prosecution so cavalierly rejects was attested by highly reliable sources. Stalin's obituary in the *New York Times*, other publications in the *Times of London* and *Life Magazine*, as well as Robert Payne's biography of Stalin, which was based on documentary sources, deserve credence. They establish that Rosa was the sister of Lazar Kaganovich, one of the leading figures in Stalin's internal circle and the only Jew in his leadership team, and they have described her amorous relationship with Stalin. It is even possible that Stalin married Rosa after Alliluyeva's death. Although his oldest son, Yakov Dzhugashvili, has denied Rosa's ties with his father and even her very existence, we should remember that his own relationship with his father was so strained and distant that he did not even know the year of his stepmother's death or the age of his half-brother Vassily. It is more than possible that he did not know about his estranged father's new marriage.

We have heard from a member of Stalin's bodyguards who was on duty on the night of November 8 and heard a gunshot coming from Ms. Alliluyeva's bedroom, and who ran into the room and found her dead on the floor by herself.

One thing that no one has denied, and several sources have confirmed, is that Stalin treated his wife abominably at the party at Marshal Voroshilov's; that she was highly upset and agitated because of it when she returned home; that she had been deeply depressed and suffered from headaches during the months prior to the party; and that she was aware of, and upset about, his attentions to other women. This, I submit, provided sufficient motivation, in a moment of anger and despair, to end it all.

I claim that Stalin's wife Nadezhda Alliluyeva committed suicide. Despite whatever other crimes Joseph Stalin committed — and we do not deny them — he did not kill his wife.

I ask that you find the defendant not guilty.

6. Jury Instructions

Members of the jury: This case is now in your hands. In a fair trial — unlike Stalin's own sham trials just for show — the defendant cannot be found guilty unless the evidence establishes his guilt beyond reasonable doubt. I ask that you examine carefully whether the evidence of Stalin's guilt (even accounting for its indirect nature) rises to this standard. The trial is now adjourned.

7. Author's Note

Our trial is over, and you, the reader, may begin your deliberations as to whose finger pulled the trigger of the pistol that killed Nadezhda Alliluyeva. Now that these events are receding into the past and the witnesses are no longer alive, this is a question that each of us must answer on our own. To me, it appears that there is some truth in both versions of events.

Even though Stalin's guilt in the murder of his wife cannot be solidly proven, his responsibility in the deaths of millions of innocent people — either by his direct orders or by the operation of the monstrous system he inherited from Lenin and subsequently perfected — has been proven beyond reasonable doubt. Villains of Stalin's caliber are judged by History, and History will pronounce the final verdict.

Yet, current polls show that more than half of Russia's population still considers Stalin a great leader and deserving of respect and admiration. What is wrong with these people? I ask myself, and cannot find the answer.

Afterword
A Different Globe: The Diary of the Immigrant Scientist

I consider myself an extremely lucky person. Fate spared me a whole lot of dreadful horrors. I avoided the Great Purges; I was born as they approached their zenith, but by the time I was an adult they were already over. Stalin's death saved me from being orphaned — it put a halt to the trial that would have ended with my father being hanged in the Red Square. It also saved me from being raped and killed in a Government-sanctioned Jewish pogrom that the Soviet authorities were allegedly planning then. Later, I was fortunate to get an excellent education in the country's best university. I am blessed with a loving husband and a daughter who is a talented artist. And my lucky stars have propelled me through space and time to reach this place called America; a place so different from my native Russia that it might as well be a different planet.

I am often asked if I miss Russia. To some extent, this book has been an attempt at an answer. Do I miss Russia? I miss my friends; I miss my native language. I express myself much more colorfully in Russian than in my monochromatic English. But do I miss Russia? Not for a moment, no. Especially not the Russia of today. After a promising interlude of a dozen years, it has begun to regress to something resembling the Russia of my Stalinist-era childhood. I don't miss a Russia where more than fifty percent of the people call Joseph Stalin a great leader. I don't miss a Russia where, once again, America is constantly slandered as an evil empire that is mired in deadly sins.

My fellow Russian immigrants and I know that America may be a different planet, but it is not Heaven. It is a country that offers opportunities to those willing to work hard. As the saying goes, if the French work to live, the Americans live to work. This reminds me of one of my favorite Russian Jewish jokes.

A Soviet Jew decides to emigrate. He comes to a government office and tells the clerk that he wants to emigrate to America. "OK," says the clerk, "come back in two days to get your passport." The man returns the next day and says that he has changed his mind: he wants to emigrate to Israel. "OK," says the clerk, "come back in two days for your passport." The man comes back the next day and says that now he wants to emigrate to Australia. The clerk, who by this time has had enough, hands him a globe and says, "Here, pick a place and tell me where you want to go, and we'll process your documents." The man spins the globe, looks at it for a long time and finally asks, "Maybe you have a different globe?"

For me and my fellow immigrants, America became a different globe. Nothing could be more alien to the Soviet totalitarian and oppressive attitude to science than the American academic environment. At the start of my American career, it even offered me *too much* freedom so that it took me a while to adjust to the newly acquired autonomy and independence.

Do you ever notice how heavy smokers often begin coughing when they get out into the open and breathe some fresh air? My friend, a former Gulag prisoner, once told me wryly during an agonizing fit of coughing that "fresh air got into my lungs." Something similar happened to me at the start of my American career in science. Metaphorically speaking, too much fresh air got into my lungs.

Emigration and immigration are very hot topics today. Each individual story has its own nuances. My road to success was long and hard. This was how my American odyssey began.

1. We Decide to Emigrate

By the late 1980s, our hopes for a new and robust civil society in the Soviet Union were dashed. Food store shelves were empty, chaos reigned, tensions ran high and ugly incidents abound. Anti-Semitic goons from the nativist group *Pamyat* (*Memory* — not to be confused with the historical, human rights society *Memorial*) threatened pogroms. They specifically targeted me and my family because of my father's and my own publications about the Doctors' Plot. I kept finding handwritten notes in our mailbox with ugly threats against myself and even against our daughter, Victoria. I did not know that my own beautician, a visceral anti-Semite, was behind these notes. She massaged my face and tinted my eyebrows and eyelashes with one hand while writing and delivering her vile screeds with the other. But what goes around comes around: her own daughter would later marry a Jew, have a child with him and emigrate to Israel!

The resurgence of the Soviet regime seemed highly probable. Many people began to see emigration as their only chance of saving themselves and their children from further decades, if not centuries, of Communism. We, too, seeing the situation as dangerous and hopeless, contacted the U.S. embassy and applied to emigrate to the United States.

To be honest, my husband had never wanted to leave Russia, and this caused so much tension between us that there was a period when we were on the brink of divorce. But the situation in the country was becoming intolerable, so he eventually agreed to emigrate.

Because my family had been persecuted during Stalin's Doctors' Plot, we were granted refugee status by the American Embassy in Moscow. For emigration-oriented Russians, this was considered a great stroke of luck. Refugee status guaranteed help from charitable organizations to facilitate the start of a new life. It was essential for someone like my husband who had no driver's license, wasn't fluent in English and was generally unprepared for emigration. However, between our daughter Victoria and myself, we almost succeeded in turning our good fortune into disaster. Our journey to the United States was as full of unexpected twists as was the rest of my life. Our family has never clung to the straight and narrow.

To begin with, while our application was pending, Victoria took matters into her own hands and emigrated to Israel. She just could not stand it in the Soviet Union any longer and did not want to wait for the American papers.

While on a visit to the States with me in 1989, Victoria took an entrance exam to the New York Academy of Arts and was accepted with a full scholarship. A week later she was accepted by The Boston University Theater School with a very generous scholarship. She eventually decided to go with the New York Academy of Arts. However, this happened in April, and classes — and her scholarships — would not begin until the end of August. She decided to return to Russia, planning to fly back to New York in August to start her classes. This turned out to be a grave mistake. The moment she crossed the Soviet border at Sheremetyevo airport, the door slammed shut behind her. The Soviet authorities denied her an exit visa to study abroad.

These days, Russian students routinely study in the United States but in 1989, when the Soviet regime was dying an agonizingly slow death, studying abroad was a privilege granted only to the offspring of high-ranking Soviet officials. Victoria was certainly not one of them. Understandably, she was beside herself. Our immigration paperwork was still being processed and at least a year from completion. She did not want to spend an extra minute in the "evil empire" if she could help it. Impatient to leave one way or another, she applied for permission to emigrate to Israel.

She had to endure the taunts, mockery and a whole host of ridiculous bureaucratic demands as she made her way through the OVIR, the Soviet counterpart to the U.S. Citizenship and Immigration Service. Only after I had threatened to announce a hunger strike on the front steps of the OVIR office in the presence of representatives of all the major world media did Victoria finally receive her exit papers.

Even then, her trials were not over. I would like to share with you the events of her last day and night in the Soviet Union.

Victoria's Driver's License. Shortly before she was scheduled to leave, Victoria passed her driving test. It took her three or four attempts; her victory was hard-won as she is not a natural driver. She was supposed to pick up her driver's license in person a week before departure, but days passed and the license was still not ready. The GAI (the Soviet DMV) knew that Victoria was emigrating because she had already surrendered her internal Soviet passport and her citizenship and used her Israeli visa as her ID.

On the last day before departure, Victoria once again made the trip to the GAI: an hour and a half one way, at a time when minutes counted. She called us from the GAI, very upset: the license was still not ready. I blew up. "Get me a supervisor's phone number!" Victoria somehow got the number and I made the call.

A Colonel N answered (he introduced himself, but I immediately forgot his name). "My daughter, Victoria Rapoport, has to fly to Israel tomorrow," I said. "She was supposed to get her driver's license a week ago but it's still not ready. Can you help her?" "*I don't help all these Rapoports, Epsteins, Kogans,*" said Colonel N. "*They should all be exterminated!*"

Dear reader, pause for a moment to let it sink in. These words were uttered by a man in uniform, seated at his desk in a government agency!

I was terrified. Forget the driver's license; it was past time to get Victoria out of that fascist lair! But this was before the age of mobile phones, so I had no way of reaching Victoria and could only wait for her to call back. In the meantime, I called a friend of mine who worked at the popular newspaper *Arguments and Facts*, told her about my conversation with Colonel N and gave her his number. My friend called the colonel, introduced herself and said, "You just got a call from Ms. Rapoport whose daughter is leaving for Israel tomorrow. She asked you to help her daughter get her driver's license that your office has been holding back. Could you tell me, verbatim, what you just told her?" After a pause, the colonel said, "I told her that her license is ready and she can pick it up at window No. 8." Victoria came home in possession of her driver's license.

The Night Before the Flight. In accordance with regulations, we went to the customs office to check in Victoria's bag. We waited in line for three or four hours, so it was late at night by the time we drove home. I drove, my husband was in the passenger seat, and Victoria sat in the back. I pulled into our courtyard and noticed a black Volga car with its lights off, parked on the right. It was unusual; black Volgas typically belonged to government offices. I passed it and headed toward our garage. The Volga turned on its high beams and followed us, blocking the way out.

I cannot describe how terrified I was, especially recalling Colonel N's words several hours before about "all these Rapoports, Epsteins and Kogans." I seriously thought they were about to open fire. "Get down!" I yelled to Victoria, who, of course, only sat up taller. We stood like that for a minute or more, trapped in front of our garage, the Volga blocking us in from behind with its high lights glaring at us. It felt like an eternity. We had to do something. I decided to sacrifice our car, put it in reverse and stomped on the gas. The Volga began to pull back. I forced it all the way back, pulled out of the courtyard and took off down the deserted Novopeschannaya street. The Volga followed us, its high beams blazing. I turned right into a little alleyway; the Volga followed. Here, I hit a deep pothole that almost cost us our lives. The car spun out, but somehow I got it back under control and raced on ahead... but to where?

I would be hard-pressed to explain how I decided to head straight into the enemy lair — the police (militia) department of our district, which was then located in the courtyard of a large apartment building. I flew there helter-skelter through alleyways and courtyards. The Volga slowed down and stopped out on the street. It was almost four in the morning. A disheveled cop with his jacket thrown negligently over his shoulders stood on the front steps, clearly expecting us. "Why are they harassing us?" I yelled, pointing to the Volga. "No one is harassing you. They are protecting you," said the disheveled cop. "Who from? We didn't ask for protection!" The cop shrugged but said nothing. "Are we free to go?" "No one's keeping you," said the cop, and we saw the black Volga pull away and disappear around the corner.

It was five in the morning when we came home. Victoria's flight was at nine. That night, her last night in the country, was like a good shot in the arm against any future homesickness...

On March 10, 1990, at the age of twenty-four, with no support system, relatives, or close friends awaiting her, Victoria left for Israel. As a result, her name was automatically dropped from the American list of refugee candidates. She had hoped to go from Israel to study in America, but unbeknownst to her, in crossing the Israeli border, she had slammed the door to the United States shut for several years.

From the moment she left, I knew no peace. Starting a new life in a different country is very difficult for anyone, and the fact that she was a young artist raised by overprotective parents didn't help. It was very difficult to reach her in Israel; telephone calls had to be scheduled a week in advance and usually for 3 or 4 am. Sometimes Victoria was not at home at the appointed time, and I would go weeks without hearing from her and would be worried out of my mind. I knew that I would never learn enough about her life while I was still in the Soviet Union and could never help her from there. For me, therefore, our own emigration was a foregone conclusion.

At that time, my chances of visiting Victoria in Israel from the Soviet Union were almost nil. Nevertheless, using a number of creative tricks, I managed to wangle a visit to Jerusalem several months after her arrival. I came to Italy at the invitation of the Italian publisher of my father's book which included my story. A friend of his, an influential Israeli living in Italy (later I realized he must have been a Mossad agent), helped me get an Israeli visa. The visa was stamped on a separate form, for geopolitical reasons, so it would not show in my Soviet passport. I used the royalties from our Italian edition to purchase plane tickets to Israel.

I found Victoria's living conditions to be desperately poor. Her room was the size of a mousehole and a broken window frame prevented the window from being closed. These seemingly unimportant details would have a direct impact on the events several months later that led to my defection to the United States.

Meanwhile, right around the time our refugee status was approved, I was invited to work as a visiting professor at the University of Utah for one semester. I saw an opportunity to prepare the way for our eventual immigration. I was reluctant to accept the charity of Jewish organizations and hoped to use my semester in America to find a permanent job. Besides, processing our refugee documents was taking too long, but the invitation to work was right there and could not wait: the semester was about to begin. I flapped my wings and flew to America on a work visa, hoping to swing by Moscow after the end of the semester to get my husband, complete the remaining paperwork and leave for good. Fate had other plans, as it often does: I did not return to Russia.

Thinking back, I am amazed at how quickly our regular, established Soviet life flew to pieces as soon as the Iron Curtain began to twitch open. In our twenty-five years together, my husband, our daughter and I had rarely spent more than a week or two apart, and they were mostly for work trips. But in the March of 1991, Victoria flew to Israel, and in August that same year I flew to America, leaving my husband alone in Moscow. From a dot on a map of Moscow we became a triangle with its points in Moscow, Jerusalem, and Salt Lake City. Because communication between these countries was difficult and unreliable at that time, I think of this triangle as one drawn with faint, dotted lines with large, yawning gaps between the dots. Years would pass before we could be reunited.

2. The Starting Point

With Gorby's *perestroika* in full swing, the restrictions on Jewish scientists traveling abroad were abolished. My work was known to Western colleagues through my publications; I had often been invited to speak at conferences abroad, but the Soviet authorities had always kept me from attending them. Now the leash was released. For the first time in fifty years, I was granted a passport to attend a scientific conference in a Western country. And what a country — Switzerland! The conference in Lausanne was followed by one in Prague. I attended both.

My presentations were well received. As a follow-up, I received numerous invitations from scientists across the globe. One of those invitations came from Professor Lawrence DeVries, the associate Dean of the College of Engineering at the University of Utah who worked in a closely related field. Dr. DeVries invited me to spend a semester at the University of Utah as a recipient of the W. W. Clyde Distinguished Chair. I happily accepted the invitation. Without waiting for the completion of my emigration formalities, on August 29, 1990 I arrived in Utah on a working visa. I was hopeful that this American work experience would help me to quickly find a job when my husband and I arrived in the USA as immigrants. As described below, life offered us more surprises; nothing worked out the way I had expected.

I enjoyed every moment of my first term in Utah. Everything was new, challenging, and exciting. I was the first Russian and the first woman to occupy the W. W. Clyde Chair, which made me almost a celebrity. I was pursued by journalists seeking interviews and gave talks at various gatherings; I was even invited to give a lecture at the very prestigious Frontiers of Science forum, to which Nobel Prize laureates have been sometimes invited. That year no Nobel laureate was on hand, and they invited me instead.

The gathering took place in a large and beautiful conference hall at the Utah Museum of Fine Arts. I was told that my lecture was intended for a broad audience and should be both scientific and popular. This did not scare me as I had extensive experience in giving these kinds of lectures in the Soviet Union. I suggested the topic "Totalitarianism and Science."

3. Totalitarianism and Science: Frontiers of Science Lecture

In my lecture, I told the audience about the fate of three Soviet women scientists: Lina Stern, Olga Lepeshinskaya, and Nina Klyuyeva.

The reader already met Lina Stern, a world-renowned physiologist, in Chapter 1. She was the first woman to be elected to the Soviet Academy of Sciences. My mother, a professor of physiology, worked closely with Lina. I grew close with Lina as well.

Lina came from a rich Jewish family in Latvia. With characteristic humor, she told me why she became a scientist. Her father arranged a debutante ball for his daughters, where her younger, more beautiful sister was a resounding success. All the most eligible young men invited the younger sister to dance, forgetting about Lina. "At that moment," Lina said, "I realized that my destiny was science." She remained devoted to science throughout the ninety years of her remarkable life and died a virgin.

Lina studied in Geneva and enjoyed an illustrious career in Switzerland, but she left everything to come to the Soviet Union in the mid-1920s, captivated by the idea of helping to build "the most progressive society on Earth."

In January 1949, Lina was arrested together with other members of the Soviet Jewish Anti-Fascist Committee which included prominent Jewish intellectuals. All of them were executed in 1952 except for Lina, who was spared and sent into exile. Stalin himself crossed out her name from the execution list. There is a theory that Stalin thought Lina possessed the secret of longevity. She spent five years in prison and in exile.

On June 2, 1953, three months after Stalin's death, Lina returned from exile to Moscow. She stayed with us because her apartment required thorough fumigation: for five years moths had feasted on Lina's Persian carpets and fur coats. During those days, Lina told my parents a lot about her years in prison and in exile. Soon she developed memory problems and forgot all about those years. My father called this, according to Ivan Pavlov, protective inhibition. Interestingly, memory problems did not interfere with Lina's scientific work. She returned to active research and my mother worked with her until Lina's death in 1968.

As a reminder, Lina was in the vanguard of scientists who studied the blood-brain barrier. She was convinced that brain diseases could be cured by injecting drugs into the spinal fluid, thus bypassing the blood-brain barrier. Under Lina's guidance, my mother and her colleagues injected the new antibiotic, streptomycin, into the spinal fluid of a girl who had acquired tuberculosis meningitis, a fatal disease. The little girl survived. This was the first such cure in the world!

At that time, streptomycin was a rare drug that had been just recently developed in the United States. Its distribution was under strict government control. Lina got hold of some streptomycin through her brother who lived in America. It is not known how he had obtained it and how he delivered it to Lina, but he got into serious trouble in America and had to move to Switzerland.

During streptomycin's early days, no one knew the correct dosage of the drug. As streptomycin affects the auditory nerve, the girl who had been treated by Lina's team lost her hearing.

While I related this story during my lecture, someone in the audience gave a loud sob. I stopped talking and peered at the audience. A woman stood up and said, "You have just told the story of my aunt. She's completely deaf but she's a prominent scientist with a Ph.D. in microbiology. She had just spent a month with me here and flew back to Moscow only yesterday. I never knew all the details of this story. Thank you!" The audience began to clap. I was stunned. My life is filled with these incredible coincidences! Some thought that I had staged this whole thing on purpose.

Olga Lepeshinskaya, author of a pseudo-scientific theory of spontaneous life generation from a mysterious "vital substance," stood at the opposite pole of the scientific world. Stalin had elevated her, along with fellow biologist Trofim Lysenko, who famously rejected genetics, to the top of the Soviet biology establishment. Lepeshinskaya had received a Stalin Prize for her "discovery" of the "vital substance."

Oddly, Lepeshinskaya had great respect for my father and visited us at our dacha to try and proselytize him, much to his amusement. She even invited my father to a party at the House of Scientists celebrating her newly awarded Stalin Prize. Moscow biologists were highly amused when my father jokingly asked this venerable septuagenarian for her hand in marriage. "Olga Borisovna," my father said, "you are now the most desirable girl in Moscow. Will you marry me, and we'll make children from the *vital substance*?" Malicious tongues wagged: they said that she was pleased with the first part of the "proposal," but not with the second.

The third name on my list in the Frontiers of Science lecture was the microbiologist *Nina Klyuyeva*, a respected scientist with a tragic story. You already met her and her husband Grigory Roskin in the chapter on Vasily Parin. This couple pioneered cancer biotherapy and developed a preparation that manifested high anti-cancer activity in tumor-bearing mice. Stalin called their development an "invaluable achievement." Klyuyeva and Roskin wrote a manuscript on their research and shared it with their American colleagues. When Stalin knew about that he got furious. However, he did not arrest the authors because he had personal interest in their research (Stalin developed lip cancer due to constant pipe smoking). Instead, he subjected Klyuyeva and Roskin to an utterly humiliating and painful public trial, the so-called "court of honor." Roskin soon died of a heart attack; Klyuyeva outlived him by seven years. Further studies eventually showed that their vaccine was ineffective on humans. Still, their work was the first ever attempt at cancer biotherapy, an important and promising field of current biomedical research.

My Frontiers of Science lecture was a resounding success. A large crowd surrounded me after I had finished, asking questions, thanking me, and inviting me for more talks. One couple waited for the crowd to disperse before they approached me to introduce themselves. Their names were Dixie and Michael Schafir, and they would later rescue me from a very difficult situation.

4. An Accidental Defector: I Stay in the U.S.

All good things must come to an end, and in late December 1990 my term as a W. W. Clyde Chair was over. I gave a farewell party and left for Moscow.

The plane from Salt Lake City to Moscow makes a stopover at the JFK airport in New York City. As luck would have it, while I was in the air, Saddam Hussein had begun pummeling Israel with rockets. The Gulf War had started and all TV monitors at JFK were showing the rockets flying and falling on Israel. A CNN panel was discussing whether the rockets contained biological, chemical, or nuclear capabilities. They reported that everyone in Israel had been given gas masks and instructed to seal their windows.

I froze in my tracks. A vision of Victoria's broken window frame flashed in my mind. The words "biological," "chemical," and "nuclear" repeated again and again by CNN commentators paralyzed me with fear for my daughter.

As I mentioned before, in the Soviet Union during this time, communication with Israel was severely restricted. I would have had to request a telephone call a week in advance and would only be allotted times in the middle of the night, at 3 or 4 in the morning. If these were the conditions in times of "peace," what could I expect in war time? Regrettably, the Soviet Union supported Saddam Hussein. No less depressing was my suspicion that the SCUD rockets falling on Israel had been developed at my own institute by my friends and colleagues in the department of Solid Explosives, next door to my department of Chemical and Biological Processes. These rockets were now flying to kill my daughter. It was too much to bear. As I walked slowly to my transfer gate, it became clear to me that if I flew to Moscow right now, I would probably never see or hear from my daughter again. By the time I arrived at the gate, I had made my decision.

"I'm not flying with you. Please give me back my bag."

The person at the desk nodded and no questions were asked. My bag, stuffed with American souvenirs for my family and friends, was returned to me, and I sat next to it on the bench at the airport. I needed to decide what to do next. Within one short minute, owing to the fear I had for my daughter, her broken window frame, and Saddam Hussein's Soviet-supplied SCUD missiles, my status had changed. From this moment on, I would be a defector.

My former student Eugene Step was at that time a postdoctoral fellow at Columbia University. He and his wife Julia had become our close family friends, so I stayed with them and spent three agonizing weeks sitting on the floor in front of the TV watching rockets fall on Israel. Once I managed to get Victoria on the phone. While we were talking, the TV in my room announced that a new series of rockets was flying to Israel. Simultaneously, I heard a siren go off on Victoria's side of the phone, and Victoria said, "Sorry, I need to go to a shelter." It was excruciating. I needed to make up my mind. I could not stay with the Steps forever, so I made calls to Moscow to talk to my husband and to my father. I told them that I had decided to stay in America because if I returned, we would probably never see or hear from Victoria again. My father said that I had made the right decision. My husband became extremely upset but did not insist on my return. In 1991, a restoration of Communist Party rule appeared very likely, which made my return to the Soviet Union even more inconceivable.

My fears were not imaginary. In August 1991 (just eight months after my defection), a group of hardliners attempted to stage a coup, kidnapping and imprisoning Mikhail Gorbachev for a few days. It seemed to spell the end of all my hopes for my husband's liberation from his cage. I knew that if the hardliners won, I would never see him again. Moreover, his life in Russia as the husband of a defector would be very hard indeed.

At the time of the coup, I was attending a scientific conference in Hungary where I was to give a presentation. All the conference participants, especially those from the former Soviet satellite countries, spent most of the time sitting with our Hungarian colleagues in front of a TV while they translated the news to us. Understandably, I could not think about anything else. But about ten minutes before my scheduled presentation, a miracle happened: the coup collapsed! I ran to the conference hall just in time to jump up onto the podium and start my scientific report with: "The coup is over! We won!" There was a squall of applause!

It is common practice at scientific conferences that presentations are rated and the winners' names are announced during the post-conference banquet. At this particular conference, the first two minutes of my presentation where I had announced the end of the coup were unanimously voted to be the absolute winner.

At the time of my defection, I still had some leftover money from my time as the W. W. Clyde Chair. Utah was the only place that I knew and liked and where I had made some friends. After three weeks with the Steps, I bought a plane ticket and returned to Utah. All this time I had been so depressed that I could not bring myself to call anybody except my husband and my father in Moscow. Just before my departure from New York, I called Michael and Dixie Schafir and asked them for help.

5. Prisoner No. 184515

Michael Schafir had a number tattooed on his arm: 184515. He was born in Poland, on the border with Germany, and had survived the Holocaust. He was twelve when he was imprisoned in a concentration camp, the only one of forty-seven family members to survive two death marches. All kinds of random people helped him survive, including a Nazi who, every day, would bring Michael a sandwich and toss it over the fence. When the Allies entered Buchenwald in April, 1945, Michael was dying of typhus. They transferred him to an American hospital and nursed him back to health. He went to school, first in Germany and then in America, and in 1955, graduated from the Tulane University School of Medicine with a degree in pediatrics.

Michael was a kind and cheerful man with wonderful, luminous eyes. He was very short, which must have helped him in his career by putting his smallest patients at ease. In addition, he turned out to have good business sense and eventually became quite wealthy. Michael always remembered that he owed his life to many people, including those whose names he would never know. After he had built his fortune, he devoted his money and energy to helping new immigrants come to America, making this his life's credo. I was fortunate to become one of his protégées.

Dixie, his second wife, grew up a Mormon but converted to Judaism and, like many neophytes, was especially passionate about helping her husband in his good deeds (in Hebrew, *mitzvot*). The night we met after my lecture, Michael and Dixie gave me their business cards and told me to call them any time if I needed help. Their offer was so sincere and heartfelt that, despite my lifelong reluctance to be a burden, I found it easy to place a call from New York to their number to say that I needed their help because I had not taken my flight to Russia and was returning to Utah.

Michael and Dixie met me at the airport and virtually adopted me. After my return from New York, I spent several months at their house and they helped me survive through the tough transitional period.

Michael's house stood high on a hill in one of the prettiest neighborhoods of Salt Lake City. The view from there onto the Great Salt Lake valley at sunset was magical. Our valley is crisscrossed by a network of roads, like a sheet of graph paper. At night, these roads transformed into double strands of rubies and diamonds: ruby-red taillights of westbound traffic and glittering diamond headlights moving east, toward us. Over to the right, a barely visible sliver of the Great Salt Lake gleamed like molten gold.

But I had no eyes for the view, preoccupied as I was with the heavy task of mastering the complex, convoluted and multifaceted art of living in mysterious America. I lacked all the essentials: a car, a driver's license, car insurance, a place to live and, most importantly, a job. I did not have the heart to call any of my former colleagues. Therefore, no one in Utah except Michael and Dixie knew that I had not made it to Moscow, was still in the U.S. and, moreover, had returned to Salt Lake City.

When I turned up at the University unannounced, it created a small stir. Although my work visa was still in effect, my term as a W. W. Clyde chair had ended and there was no more funding for me. To my colleagues' credit, within two weeks they unanimously approved me for the position of a research professor. To be honest, this cost them nothing because a research professorship is not a salaried position, nor does it support students or subordinates. I was expected to fund all of these things myself through grants. The only thing this position entitled me was the right to apply for grants in the name of the University of Utah.

Dixie and Michael were almost impossibly kind. They drove me to the University every day and, later, organized their neighbors so that someone would drop me off and someone else would pick me up.

While living with Dixie and Michael, I was looking for a cheap apartment so that I could relieve the Schafirs of the heavy burden of hosting me. The story of how I tried to rent my first apartment in America deserves its own chapter.

6. I Try to Rent an Apartment

I was looking through the classifieds when I came across an ad for a remarkably cheap apartment in a good neighborhood. I called the number and the owner or manager said I could come see it at any time as his agent lived in the same building. The agent turned out to be a massive square boulder of a man with a repulsive face. The building was divided into two apartments by a thin drywall partition; the agent lived in the other apartment. I looked over the apartment and liked it; it even had a mountain view from a side window. The only problem was that there was no sink or tub in the bathroom, only a stinking puddle in the middle of the floor. "We're getting the bathroom fixed after our last renters moved out," said the agent. "Tomorrow it will all be fixed. By the way, where is your accent from?" I told him. "All of Russia's problems started when Stalin died," said my future neighbor. I was stunned: "Do you know that Stalin caused the deaths of twenty million innocent people?" "First of all, it wasn't twenty million, it was only seven. [*"Only" seven million! — NR.*] These are KGB numbers, and I believe them. Second, what if you had a choice that tomorrow your family would die, or twenty million strangers would die — which would you choose?" I was enraged: "I think if I had a choice of who should die, I would pick the person asking me such questions."

I ran to a telephone and called my friend and colleague Joel Dubao. I had become friends with him and his family during my term as the W. W. Clyde Chair; Joel had even taught me to drive his car. I told him about my conversation with my neighbor-to-be. "I don't think I should rent this apartment." "You don't understand how American privacy works," said Joel. "You'll never see your neighbor again after you sign the lease. Do you like the apartment? Then take it!" Joel had been born and raised in this country while I was a newcomer, so I trusted his experience and advice. The agent took me to his apartment to sign the lease. The first thing I noticed was the big revolver on his desk. "Do I need to buy a gun like this if I rent this place?" I asked. "It's enough that I have one," said the agent in all seriousness.

I signed the lease, paid the deposit and the first month's rent, and received the keys. With Joel's help, I moved in with my meager belongings, donated by the Clyde family and by Dixie and Michael and some other friends after my return to Utah. These things — a bed with bedding, a table, two chairs, a pretty table lamp — had been stored for me in Joel's basement.

That same evening, I flew out to visit some friends, expecting the bathroom to be fixed in the meantime. When I returned a few days later, the bathroom was unchanged. There was still no sink or tub and the puddle in the middle of the floor was even more odorous. I ran to the University and called the owner: "What's going on? Your agent told me that the bathroom would be fixed the day after the lease was signed but it's still not fixed! I can't live there!" "Why not?" asked the owner, "I know all about you. They don't shower every day where you come from." I gasped at such rudeness. "You're quite wrong. I shower every day, sometimes twice a day. I'm afraid I can't live in your apartment." "Great! You and people like you come to America and steal our jobs. You should be deported; I will make sure you are." Like a bad smell, the old memory of my Russian experiences came to me. Was it really all the same in America? I hung up and called Joel, crying. He became very serious and said, "I'm calling the police. You should come outside in 20 minutes. I will pick you up and we will go get your money and your things."

Joel came to get me dressed in camouflage and armed to the teeth. Seeing him like this scared me more than talking to that bastard. I asked, "Why are you armed?" Joel replied, "You don't know these people. A police car will be waiting for us on the corner of your street and will drive up with us."

There was indeed a police car waiting at the corner of my street. Joel honked his horn and the policeman turned on his flashers and pulled up in front of us like a flagship. In the dark, we saw two figures at my door tossing my things out on the ground. At the sight of a police car, they became meek as mice: "Sir, the lady said she didn't want to live here, so we thought we would help her move out her things." "It looks to me like you're throwing them out, not moving them out," said the policeman. "Will you return her money and cancel the lease?" "Of course, like we told her!" "Then bring her check back, or if you have already deposited it, write her another one." "Certainly, sir; right away, sir!" Joel, in the meantime, was loading my things into his car. I was sorry to see that the beautiful antique lamp that looked like a Greek amphora, a gift from the Clydes, had been shattered. "You can sue them for damages and mental distress," said the policeman. "If you choose to do so, I will prepare a statement." "No, I just want to get my money back and get out of here as soon as possible," I said.

Now, having lived in America for about thirty years, on hindsight I probably should have sued them and won significant damages, but back then, new and alone, that was the last thing on my mind. I stayed in Joel's basement for a while until I found another apartment.

Time passed — probably about a year — and April 20 came around. That year, the local Nazis held a march in front of our state Capitol to mark the anniversary of Hitler's birth. A local newspaper published a large photograph of the march. In the first row, sporting swastika armbands, marched my erstwhile neighbor and the owner or manager of that building. My first foray into the American real estate market had almost landed me in a Nazi lair.

We learned later that the Nazis and the white supremacists had a nest in the south of Utah, in Zion National Park. They had chosen that site on purpose; they called themselves the "true children of Zion" — not to be confused with the Jews who, according to them, were not the true children of Zion and should therefore be kicked out of Zion and destroyed. The "true children of Zion" were equal opportunity racists who hated all minorities (especially colored ones). That was their downfall. Under American law, people are free to think all sorts of hateful things but not to act upon them. The white supremacists were evicted from the national park in full accord with the Constitution, whereupon their whole crew went north and settled in the neighboring state of Idaho. One day, they verbally and physically assaulted a Native American man walking past their camp and were arrested (I would not be surprised if the Native American had been sent by the police). The leader of the white supremacists was put on trial and given a lengthy prison sentence (he later died in prison), the group's property was confiscated, and their time in our parts came to an end.

7. The Ordeal

The start of my new life in America was an extremely difficult time for me. I did not know how the grant system worked, my difficulties with the English language were very real, and I was still learning my way around computers (I got my first computer in 1990 when I was awarded the W. W. Clyde Chair; Dr. DeVries had to teach me how to turn it on and off and how to use a mouse). My only assets at the time were my excellent education and some scientific ideas that I hoped to pursue.

At first, I survived through substitute teaching, taking those classes that tenured professors did not want to teach. For pennies, I taught classes that came along without knowing if the class would be offered again the following semester. There were a couple of periods when there were no classes for me to teach. Hence, I went without payment for several months at a time, unable to even apply for unemployment benefits because, as a research professor, I was considered employed. It was an exhausting time for me, full of worry and insecurity. One needed nerves of steel to avoid sinking into despair.

While teaching, I did my best to stay aware of what my fellow researchers were doing, trying to figure out how one went about getting research grants in America. And my fellow researchers were doing amazing things. One day someone took me to see a calf who had received an artificial heart implant the previous year. The calf, sleek and clean, was chewing contentedly and generally looking great.

You may recall that the first artificial heart implantation in a human, the famous Jarvic-7, had been performed at the University of Utah in the early 1980s. Even Soviet TV carried the story of Barney Clark, the first recipient of that device. At that time, the artificial heart was a massively huge machine, weighing something like 400 kg (or was it lbs.?). Barney Clark lived only a few months with the device, but the second recipient lived almost two years. Since then, the device itself and the size and weight of related equipment have continued to improve under the leadership of my University of Utah colleague, the brilliant Danish researcher Wilhelm Kolb, a pioneer in the field of artificial organs. Artificial hearts have become the norm today with many people around the world living with the device, but when I arrived in the early 1990s, researchers were only halfway toward modern prototypes and I was privileged to witness and admire the revolution that was taking place before my eyes.

Of course, the artificial heart is just one part of the general field of artificial organs. The biomedical engineering program at the University of Utah was working on things that used to be the province of science fiction, such as artificial hands that obeyed brain signals like their natural counterparts, artificial eyes, visual prosthetics for the blind, and so forth. Here at the University of

Utah, novel scientific ideas were no longer mere fiction and con-
jectures but pure, glorious science.

I felt unmoored observing this new world. All that I had
done in science until then suddenly seemed gray, flat, boring, and
unworthy. True science was happening right here at the Department of Biomedical Engineering. My life was beginning anew
and I was ready to jettison all my previous experience in order to
become part of this amazing new world.

8. A Happy Encounter

Fortunately, I did not have to jettison my entire past. By a happy
accident, some of my work experience from the Moscow Institute of Chemical Physics — experience that had no equivalent in
Utah — turned out to be a good fit for one of the artificial organ
projects. The head of the project, the granddaughter of Svante
Arrhenius (a great Swedish chemist and one of the first recipients
of the Nobel prize), would soon become a close friend of mine.

We met by pure accident. During a scientific conference
in Salt Lake City, I found myself at dinner seated next to a nice
woman of about my age. She knew about me and my W. W. Clyde
professorship, but I had never seen her before. We introduced ourselves: Karin Caldwell; Natasha Rapoport. In the middle of small
talk, Karin said in passing, "When my grandfather got his Nobel
Prize…" I sat up: "Your grandfather got a Nobel Prize?" I was
clearly the only one at our table not to know this. "Yes," said Karin,
"my grandfather was Svante Arrhenius. Do you know this name?"

I was stunned. In my prior life at the Institute of Chemical
Physics in Moscow, I had probably said the name of Svante Arrhenius at least five times a day — the Arrhenius equation, the Arrhenius plot, the Arrhenius energy of activation, his theory of ionic

dissociation; all these concepts were an integral part of my typical work day. But I had never wondered about the origin of the name, assuming that Arrhenius was like Archimedes or Pythagoras, a man from centuries long gone. After all, he was a classic, like Newton or Avogadro, but here I was sitting next to his granddaughter, who had probably bounced on his lap!

Karin was pleased, and our conversation gained serious traction. She told me that Henry Eyring (number two in my pantheon of chemical kinetics) had worked at the U of U chemistry department until recently. Karin's husband had studied under him. I told Karin that Eyring's 1941 book, *The Theory of Rate Processes* (which he had co-authored with Samuel Glasstone and Keith Laidler), had been translated into Russian and was one of my favorite books on chemical kinetics, and that I had even brought it with me to Utah.

In turn, Karin told me that Henry Eyring had been a Mormon and had married a Mormon woman who refused to leave Utah. Karin further elaborated that had he worked at Princeton, for example, he probably would have won a Nobel Prize. He was nominated and short-listed for the prize, but the night before the prizes were announced he stayed up till morning waiting for a call from Sweden that never came. Henry Eyring had recently passed away, and now one of his sons worked at the Chemistry department.

The University of Utah suddenly took on new colors for me. If people like Henry Eyring or Wilhelm Kolb worked there, it was certainly the place to be.

"And what do you do, Natasha?" asked Karin. I told her about the Moscow Institute of Chemical Physics, about its director, Nikolay Semyonov (our own Nobel Prize laureate), and about my prior work. I also explained how I happened to be in Utah. Then I asked her what she did.

Karin was working on preventing the rejection of implanted artificial organs, trying to make their surface biologically compatible with the host tissue. This idea was new to me. Here it is in short. If, after the implantation, a protein molecule from the host body that is deposited on the implant surface changes its shape, it signals to the body that a foreign object is present. This triggers an immune response that results in rejection. To prevent rejection, protein adsorption to the implant surface should be inhibited. To accomplish this, the surface of the artificial organ is covered with a protective layer comprised of special long molecules, which suppresses the adsorption of proteins. Although this strategy has been shown to work, the optimal structure of the protective layer has not yet been found. Scientists do not know whether it is best to arrange the long molecules in a long and tight brush-like formation or to leave them to oscillate more loosely, like seaweed on the ocean floor. These two strategies are more or less mutually exclusive: the molecules arranged in a tight brush can only move around with difficulty, like passengers in a crowded bus.

It occurred to me that I could help solve this dilemma. My heart skipped a beat at the realization that this could be my lucky stroke. I told Karin that this was in my wheelhouse and I may have a solution.

I knew of a method to measure the motion rate of long molecules, which had been developed in the USSR but was rarely used in the United States. I could measure the motion of molecules in the protective layer and correlate it with protein adsorption to find the optimal structure that would prevent adsorption.

Karin immediately caught on with my idea and became very excited. She had a tiny amount left on one of her grants and offered it to me. To me, this was manna from heaven: my first American research project. This project would eventually prove to be my pivot toward oncology, where, years later, I would be developing a new technique for the targeted delivery of anti-cancer drugs into tumors.

9. A "Magic Bullet"

The concept of a drug that could hit its target without damaging healthy tissues was first formulated by Paul Ehrlich, a Nobel Prize laureate in medicine, more than a century ago. He called his concept a "magic bullet." In medicine, directing a drug exclusively to a desired site of action is called targeting.

No other field of medicine could benefit more from drug targeting than cancer chemotherapy, which is known to be plagued by severe side effects. Unfortunately, the development of a "magic bullet" has been fraught with difficulties. After decades of active research in academia and industry, we are still not quite there.

Various approaches toward achieving this goal have been investigated. The technique that I suggested was based on the development of tiny drug-carrying particles that retained the drug after injection but released it locally into the tumor under the action of tumor-directed ultrasound.

We manufactured tiny drug-loaded droplets, called nanodroplets, that could convert into bubbles under the action of ultrasound, as if one was blowing tiny balloons. During the droplet-to-bubble conversion, the drug would be locally released from the particle and internalized by tumor cells.

We tested this technology in mice bearing breast, ovarian, or pancreatic cancer and derived spectacular results. This eventually brought me several patents and major grants from the National Cancer Institute. In 2007, my paper on the subject was featured in the *Journal of National Cancer Institute* and made quite a stir in the biomedical world, spreading from the USA, Canada, and

Europe to India, Malaysia, and South Africa. There was a lot of interest in this technology from venture capitalists, although, unfortunately, this has not yet come to pass for reasons beyond me. I was unable to begin human trials of my technology before my retirement in 2012, but my work is continued and extended through my younger colleagues. Hopefully, they will bring it to a successful conclusion in clinical applications soon.

Everything described above came many years after my arrival to the USA. I worked literally day and night. This superhuman effort gave me my sorely needed American work experience. Five years after my arrival, I got the first grant of my own. It was short — just for one year — but very prestigious, since only 22 such grants were given nationwide. The University of Utah received a commendation from the director of the National Science Foundation, and during this year I finally had a salary I could live on. With this first grant, my life settled into the regular pattern of an American researcher, with its exhausting work and constant search for more grants.

Looking back, I can see a whole series of happy accidents and coincidences, as though a strong and kind hand was guiding me throughout my American career.

In one of these remarkable coincidences, I was invited to a party organized by the President of the University at his house for the research faculty. The Vice President for Research, Dr. Richard Koehn, a tall, handsome and imposing man who looked like the captain of a big ocean liner, stood at the door greeting guests. I had not met him before. Noticing my nametag, he asked me where I was from. I explained that I had emigrated from Russia. He said, "I am just reading a very interesting book written by your namesake, Yakov Rapoport. The book is about the Doctors' Plot in Russia. Have you ever heard about this book?" I told him I knew it very well indeed and he was really amazed by the coincidence. Dick Koehn and his wife, Sherry, became our good family friends, making my and my husband's life in America infinitely more exciting. In this unforeseen way, the publication of my father's book in the USA brought me so much more than the royalties from Harvard University Press.

Because America measures success mostly in dollars and disdains false modesty, I will mention that before my retirement, my work brought the University of Utah $3.3 million dollars, including a special award from the Director of the National Cancer Institute.

10. My Family's "Acculturation"

All of us refer to my husband, Vladimir, by his last name of Veisberg, himself included. By staying in America after the completion of my first term in Utah instead of returning to the Soviet Union, I had locked him in his Soviet cage. His American entry papers were all in order, but the trouble was on the Soviet side. It took us a lot of effort and more than a year after my defection for him to join me in the United States.

He was mentally exhausted by the time he made it to Utah. He spent his first two weeks cooped up in the darkened kitchen of my tiny apartment and I could not convince him to step outside. Eventually, he got over it and we went grocery shopping together. It should be noted that the Russia Veisberg left behind in 1991 was hunger-stricken, impoverished, and devastated, and he had never been to any other country. The American supermarket I took him to was a shock to his system. For my part, I had also experienced it before — that physical sense of nausea and dizziness at the sudden overabundance of choice — first in Hungary and then in Switzerland. After that, American malls and supermarkets no longer troubled me, but they crushed poor Veisberg like an avalanche. He nearly lost his mind; after all, back in Moscow at that time, even toilet paper was scarce.

But he liked what he saw. A month or so after our first trip to the supermarket, I decided to do an experiment and brought Veisberg to the toilet paper aisle where I innocently asked him which color and pattern of toilet paper he thought would best match our bathroom's color scheme. Veisberg began to seriously contemplate and discuss this nonsense. I gave him a look and he caught himself: "Oh, my! What's wrong with me?" "Nothing," I said, "it's OK. Hello, Mr. American!"

Of course, it was not all smooth sailing. Finding ourselves, as it were, on a different planet with a different gravity, we were bound to stumble occasionally. For my part, I thought our smoke detector was connected directly to the fire department and that we sent a signal there when it went off after Veisberg had started cooking pork chops in an overheated frying pan. The smoke detector began to howl, causing me to imagine its counterpart at the fire department howling just like that and a fire truck pulling up and slapping us with a bill that I would never finish paying off. I ran to the phone and dialed 911.

"My address is such and such. I'm calling to say that we don't have a fire, don't send a fire truck!"

"Is there a fire in your home?"

"No, there is no fire!"

"Then why are you calling?"

"I'm calling to say that there is no fire, don't send a fire truck!"

"Have you put the fire out?"

"No, there was never any fire!"

"Then why are you calling?"

"Because there is no fire!"

"But there *was* a fire?"

"No, there wasn't! My husband burned a frying pan, that's all!"

"Then why are you calling?"

We went around in circles five or six times while preventing some other poor souls who may have really needed urgent help from getting through. That was how I learned that our smoke detector was not actually connected to the fire department.

Soon after joining me in Utah, Veisberg began to attend "acculturation" classes, learning to speak and to drive, and also learning about American customs. He was 62 and found his studies challenging, especially with the English language, but any small improvement looks impressive when one starts from zero. And he was really making progress. Eventually he decided that he had mastered it all and quit the class. He now could communicate at the supermarket. More importantly, he had a driver's license, having passed his driving test on his first try — unlike me, who had driven for over 20 years back in Moscow but had failed the American test twice due to my bad Russian driving habits.

However, having quit school, Veisberg became bored doing nothing at home and unhappy being dependent on me. It was demeaning and depressing to him, so he began looking for work, and then work found him. A responsible, reliable, hard-working and charming man, he was offered a full-time job as a maintenance man at the Salt Lake City synagogue. Of course, this was a far cry from his former job as a department head at the Moscow Institute of Electrical Thermal Equipment, but he accepted it gladly and his mood improved noticeably. Although temporary, work cheered Veisberg up immensely and he was himself once again.

And then, finally, our daughter Victoria and her husband Michael came from Israel. As I had explained earlier, Victoria had hoped to go from Israel to study in America, but it became apparent that once she had set foot on Israeli soil, the doors of American schools were closed to her. Evidently, there was some informal agreement between Israel and America that new immigrants to Israel (*olim*) were not allowed into America until they had adapted and established deep roots in Israel. Although the New York Academy of Art kept renewing her stipend for several years in a row, the U.S. consulate in Jerusalem constantly declined her a visa. Nothing helped; not requests from the director of the New York Academy of Art to the U.S. consul in Israel, not my tearful entreaties, not even letters from Senator Orrin Hatch. Evidently, Victoria's file had landed on the desk of some clerk who was determined to defend, to the death, America's shores from her. Instead of studying at the New York Academy of Art, Victoria worked as a cleaning lady at a hotel and a nursing assistant at a retirement home.

What finally helped was another one of those happy coincidences. One evening, the phone rang in my Salt Lake City apartment. A pleasant male voice addressed me in slightly accented English. He introduced himself as Adrian, a professor in the theater department of our university. He was intending to stage a play that semester based on Mikhail Bulgakov's novel, *The Master and Margarita*. He would love it if I could talk to his students about the Russian life depicted in the novel and wondered if I could stop by the theater department that Saturday and chat with his students for an hour. He warned me that his students were woefully ignorant of literature and history in general, not only their Russian varieties. I wondered how he himself had come to be so well informed but did not probe further. When I met him, Adrian turned out to be a Romanian Jew who had escaped across the border into Austria, in the middle of the night, at significant risk to his life from trigger-happy border guards on either side. He explained, "I couldn't live there any longer under Chaushesku. I couldn't breathe there. I thought, if they shoot me, then so be it, but at least I have a chance of making it across. And I did!" From Austria, Adrian went on to Israel. A theater director by training, he worked odd jobs until he met a charming American tourist from Utah and went to America with her.

Only a man who had lived through the horrors of a Socialist regime could have turned *The Master and Margarita* into such a brilliant play. As we agreed, I came to the theater department at 2 pm to spend an hour with his students. At 1 am the following morning, we were still sitting on the floor and talking to the students about Russia and Mikhail Bulgakov, about life here and back there, about nothing in particular. The students asked me lots of questions, to which I did not always have an answer. We became instant friends. From that moment and until the opening day of the show, I attended every rehearsal as both audience and consultant. Rehearsals began in the evening and often ran far into the night. That was a happy time for me. Once again, I experienced the creative atmosphere I had left behind in Moscow and had missed so much.

Halfway to the premiere, I finally mustered the courage to show Adrian Victoria's old theater sketches I had with me in Utah and tell him about her immigration troubles. First, Adrian was struck by Victoria's work, and then he scolded me: "Why didn't you tell me before? Your daughter is a great artist! We'll get her out of there!" Adrian was indeed familiar with the problem of immigrating from Israel to America: "It's almost impossible for *olim* to get a student visa but a work visa is much easier. I am going to send her an invitation from the University to work on *The Master and Margarita*. I hope it works."

It worked. Victoria got a work visa and her husband Michael received a visa as her accompanying spouse.

To my great chagrin, *The Master and Margarita* turned out to be Adrian's last show in Utah. He got invited to work in New York, which was not surprising since he was a very talented director. *The Master and Margarita* was a runaway success, beyond anything a student production could expect. People flocked to see it.

In Salt Lake City, Victoria came to the attention of George Maxwell, the chief set designer of a municipal theater company and a great theatrical artist decorated with a Tony award. George hired Victoria as his assistant and they worked together for several years at the theater and at the renowned Shakespeare Festival. Maxwell included Victoria's works and name in his own art exhibitions and later organized two solo shows of her etchings.

But all good things must come to an end, and so did Victoria's work visa, raising the eternal question of what to do next. At Maxwell's advice, Victoria enrolled in the Master's program at our theater department and finally received the student visa she had so long been denied. I must stress that the University never had reason to regret it. Victoria earned both first prizes (in costume and set design) among graduates of theater arts programs of the Western states and a second place nationwide. Not only were her works exhibited at the Kennedy Center, but Broadway theaters seemed to be within her reach. But as I said before, our family never does things the normal way. Having pocketed her high prizes, Victoria declared that she no longer wanted to work in theater as she felt that she would be miserable all her life if she were to do so: "The theater is like a Soviet collective farm. If the director is bad or the actors are poor, all my work will be for nothing no matter how great my costumes or decorations might be. I want to be the master of my own art. I want to pursue printmaking."

In America, people are free to stay in school for as long as they want, be they twenty, fifty, or a hundred years old. Victoria went back to school, this time in the printmaking program at the art department of the University of Illinois at Urbana-Champaign. This proved to be an excellent choice: she currently enjoys a great career as a professor and graphic artist in residence at the University of Nebraska. Her works are shown around the world, including America, Europe and Asia.

11. Barefoot on Burning Coals: Our Path to Citizenship

Veisberg was the first among us to become an American citizen. He had no trouble at all with his fingerprints, English, or citizenship test. In contrast, I, who had come to America a year before him, did not get my citizenship until much later. After half a century of working with acids and bases in chemistry labs, my fingers could not produce the clear prints required for the citizenship application. I spent two years waiting to hear back about my application and wondering what was going on. The local immigration office advised me to escalate the matter to the top, where a nice female voice told me on the phone that my fingerprints looked as though I had had plastic surgery performed on them. I was astounded:

"Plastic surgery on fingers? Who would do such a thing?"

The lady sounded surprised at my naïveté:

"What do you mean? Criminals trying to hide their tracks, of course."

"But I'm not a criminal! You have my police clearance saying that I'm clean!"

"That's true, but it only covers your time in America. We also need to know that you don't have a criminal record in your country of origin."

What a mess. I wondered which Russian agency this high American office had been talking to. If they had contacted the KGB, I was toast. I was a defector and the KGB had quite a file on me. Unwilling to wait until the two agencies finished talking, I wrote to Senator Orrin Hatch asking for his help. The University sent a letter in support of my request and, soon, a high-level fingerprinting specialist flew to Utah specifically to take my fingerprints. He was a silent, dour man with a metal band around his head bearing a big magnifying glass, like a third eye. He looked like a watchmaker or a jeweler, except that when he was working, he bore a resemblance to Cyclops. He spent a long time on my fingers, studying each print through his magnifying glass, discarding them and repeating the process until, two hours later, a perfect set of ten fingerprints and two palm prints lay before him. Only then did he look up at me and say, "You should be fine now; the prints are good." He was right; two weeks later, I got a letter stating that my application had been approved. I was finally summoned to take my citizenship test.

Unbeknownst to me, my examiner was the head of our local INS. The local branch was staffed primarily with Latinos, but the director was Caucasian. He was supposed to ask me a certain number of standard questions and hear an equal number of equally standard answers. He was visibly bored, so I decided to entertain him by showing off my erudition. One of the standard test questions is: "Can you become the President of the United States?" with the standard answer being: "No, because I was not born in this country." Being native born is, in fact, only but one of three preconditions; the President also must be over thirty-five and must have lived in America for at least fourteen years in total. As such, I answered this question as follows: "No, because first of all, I wasn't born here, and second, I'm not yet thirty-five!" The examiner perked up and smiled. He asked me if I would be keen to speak at the citizenship ceremony.

I agreed to speak and told them a true story from more than half a century ago. When I was in first grade, my whole class went to see a theater play about the horrors of American orphanages. American orphans were deprived of adequate food, dressed in rags, rapped on the knuckles with a ruler in class, and forced to listen to terrible lies about the Soviet Union. I cried throughout all three acts of the play. When I came home, I begged my parents to adopt at least one American orphan to spare him or her the awful fate I had just witnessed. My parents, normally so compassionate, unaccountably turned a deaf ear to my pleas, which rather shocked me at the time. And now, although we never did adopt an American child, America had "adopted" me. I finished my story to resounding applause and the head of the INS remembered me.

This literally saved us a year later when disaster struck, costing us all manner of untold pain and stress.

Once he became a citizen, Veisberg immediately applied for a green card for Victoria on the grounds of family reunification. His application slowly moved through the system. About five years later, it had reached the top of the pile and was granted. Now it was Victoria's turn to go to the INS with the necessary papers, which would start a new clock running and confer on her a new and better immigration status. But instead of the piece of paper conferring the new status, Victoria came home with a big red stamp in her passport that read: "ILLEGAL IMMIGRANT." Underneath, a legend in smaller font said that if she did not leave the country within seven days, she would be deported in handcuffs with no right of re-entry.

We were stunned! We felt completely lost and disoriented and could not understand what had just happened. Victoria was a full-time student, had worked at the theater for a whole year and drawn a salary through the university. How was all this possible if she was illegal?

The answer was terribly simple. The university, through a stupid oversight, had failed to renew Victoria's student visa. Every summer, Victoria submitted her application for a visa renewal to the appropriate office at the university, which then sent it to the INS. She had done it this year as well, but because her husband Michael was now also in the system and their last names were the same, some of Victoria's papers had ended up in his file and had been archived, since Victoria and Michael had separated and he had left Utah. As a result, Victoria's application had been left incomplete and was not sent on to the INS, but the university never alerted Victoria or her art department to it. With her student visa canceled, Victoria had been unknowingly walking around campus as an illegal immigrant. This was not only a disaster for us but also a big problem for the university. The university commenced evasive maneuvers to cover their backside and, despite my tearful pleas, refused to write a letter to the INS explaining the situation. Instead, they sent us to a Utah state government official in charge of foreign student visas.

He turned out to be a mean and dimwitted little man with eyes that showed little expression or emotion. He did not let us say a word but began screaming right away: "You're an illegal immigrant — get out of this country!" While we watched, he sent off a fax to the immigration enforcement team instructing them to come to our home on the date stamped on Victoria's passport and remove her in handcuffs if she had not left the country by then. And if she were not found at home, they would put her on a wanted criminals list, to be imprisoned when caught and then deported... These people did not care that she was a straight-A student, the pride of her department, or an award-winning artist with her own art shows. Instead, they treated her as if she was driving around in stolen cars, dealing drugs and shooting illegal weapons.

The clock was ticking. We knew we needed to find a good immigration lawyer, but we did not know of any. If Victoria were to leave the country, she had no place to go. There was nothing for her in Israel, since all her friends had left, and also nothing in Russia where she was no longer a citizen, having been stripped of her citizenship (as was the rule back then) on her departure to Israel. Worst of all, her name was already on file with the INS as an illegal immigrant, so if she were to leave, she would not be allowed to return. All our hopes and plans — our whole life — had been shattered in an instant, all because of some idiot who had misfiled some papers! A stupid detail, this trivial little oversight, was threatening to upend Victoria's whole life.

We racked our brains for a solution and finally, for lack of a better idea, went back to the local INS office. We had two days left. The Mexican staff kept us waiting while they helped crowds of Latino applicants. Finally, our turn came, and we were seen, as it turned out, by the same official who had stamped Victoria's passport as an illegal. Given my dealings with him before, I knew not to expect any sympathy. True to form, he was exceedingly nasty to us and threatened severe penalties if Victoria continued to trample the American soil with her illegal feet two days from now.

I was in tears, begging him to let us see a manager. The inner workings of the INS were hidden by sturdy walls and protected by locked doors, but then Fate intervened again: a door opened and my citizenship examiner walked out! He saw me crying and came over to ask what was wrong. I tried to tell him about my daughter who was about to be deported for no good reason, just because the university had neglected to renew her visa, and she — a straight-A student with lots of awards — had come in to get her green card only to discover that the gentleman over there had stamped her passport as illegal, and I really needed to speak to a manager because none of these people will listen to me, and I only have a day and a half left.

During my tearful tirade, he recognized me. "You're an American citizen now," he said. "Yes, I am, and so is my husband. We both are citizens." "Let me see your daughter's passport." He took Victoria's passport, took out a pen, crossed out the red stamp and signed his name. Only then did I realize that he was that top manager I had requested to see! "You should go right away and see Mr. X [our red-headed devil], show him this document and make sure he sends a fax canceling the forced removal order."

Afraid to believe our luck, we raced to see Mr. X who scowled when he heard our news. I made sure I saw him send the cancel-lation fax.

No matter how long I have left to live on this earth, I am con-vinced that I lost at least ten years to that red stamp in Victoria's passport. It took a toll on Victoria's health, too. I shudder to think what might have become of us if that top manager had not walked out through that door at the right moment — if he had been away, or out sick, or working in his office focused on his files… But walk out he did, and for that I am eternally grateful to our guardian angel.

And so, after all the upheavals, through a series of miracles, our family was finally reunited and normal life began — ordinary life with all its ordinary ups and downs. The years galloped past like a herd of wild horses we once saw racing by in a wild Utah prairie.

In 1998, I published my first book of memoirs (in Russian) — a notable event in our family's life (by today, I have five books

278 Stalin and Medicine: Untold Stories

published in Russian). Soon after that, I received my first $1M research grant from the National Cancer Institute, another milestone.

Victoria achieved a tenured position — a full professor at the art department of the University of Nebraska. She is an extraordinarily talented artist, as evidenced by her many art shows and high prizes.

At my husband's 85th birthday, some friends of ours gave us a wonderful gift: a clock that runs *backwards*. We try our best to tune our biological clocks accordingly.

***

I wrote in the Preface that those generations that don't know history are vulnerable to social tragedies. It appears that stories of the past are resurfacing in Russia and other countries today. I can only hope that books like this one will help prevent new tragedies.

Glossary

Alliluyeva, Nadezhda was the second wife of Joseph Stalin. The couple married in 1919 when Stalin was a 41-year-old widower and she was just eighteen. Alliluyeva and Stalin had two children: Vassily, born in 1921, and Svetlana, born in 1926. Alliluyeva studied at the Industrial Academy but never graduated, dying tragically under suspicious circumstances several weeks before the end of the program she attended. At the time of her death, her relationship with Stalin was deteriorating; according to her close friend, Polina Zhemchuzhina, the two argued frequently. Amongst other things, Alliluyeva spoke out against the purges of her fellow students at the Academy, which were carried out by Nikita Khrushchev, then Secretary of the Industrial Academy's Communist Party cell. These purges were conducted under Stalin's orders, which were aimed at ridding the school of "Mensheviks and Trotskyites." Many of Alliluyeva's friends disappeared forever in NKVD cellars.

On the night of November 8, 1932, Stalin publicly insulted his wife in front of a number of friends at a party celebrating the 15th anniversary of the October Revolution. Alliluyeva left the party accompanied by her friend Polina Zhemchuzhina. The next morning, Nadezhda Alliluyeva was found dead in her bedroom.

Bukharin, Nikolay Ivanovich was a prominent leader of the Communist International (Comintern). After Lenin's death in 1924, Bukharin became a full member of the Politburo. For a period of time, Bukharin was allied with Stalin, but in January 1937, Stalin arrested him and had him expelled from the Communist Party for being a "Trotskyite." In March 1938, he was a defendant in the last public purge trial, falsely accused of counter-revolutionary activities and espionage, found guilty, and executed.

Kaganovich, Lazar Moyseyevich was one of Stalin's closest associates. When he died in 1991 at the age of 97, he was the last surviving Old Bolshevik. The Soviet Union itself outlived him by a mere five months. Here is an excerpt from Kaganovich's obituary published in the *New York Times* on July 26, 1991:

> *"Lazar Moyseyevich Kaganovich, one of Stalin's closest aides and the last surviving Bolshevik leader...Once a towering figure in Kremlin politics, Kaganovich sometimes was regarded as the No. 2 man in the Soviet Union because of his ties to Stalin. With Stalin having turned against and liquidated so many of his associates, Kaganovich stands out in Bolshevik history for surviving at the dictator's side longer than anyone. His survival was all the more remarkable because he was the only Jew to hold high office in Stalin's final years in power. Many Jews were being arrested or purged from office, and Stalin was considering a campaign to exterminate Jews when he died in 1953. One explanation may be that Kaganovich's sister, Rosa, was believed to be intimately involved with Stalin. Some biographers have said she became his third wife, though Stalin's daughter from his second marriage has denied the reports about the woman."*

Kamenev, Lev Borisovich (born Rozenfeld) was a prominent Soviet politician. He was probably the most tragic figure in the cohort of Old Bolsheviks. He conditionally supported the Russian Provisional Government, the only democratic government in all of Russia's history, which took power in February 1917 and opposed the armed revolt carried out by the Bolsheviks under the leadership of Vladimir Lenin on October 25, 1917 (according to the Julian calendar), which became known as the October Revolution. Nevertheless, he joined the uprising, becoming one of the seven members of the first Politburo and holding a position equivalent to the Head of State in the first Soviet government. When Lenin became ill in 1922, Kamenev, together with Grigory Zinovyev and Joseph Stalin, formed a triumvirate (*troika*) that took control of the Communist Party. Kamenev was instrumental in helping Stalin retain his pre-eminent position of General Secretary of the Communist Party, in defiance of Lenin's "testament" written shortly before Lenin's death demanding Stalin's demotion. Ironically, by so doing, Kamenev sealed his own fate and that of his whole family.

Lenin's testament, which he intended to be read out at the Party Congress in April, 1923, was instead kept secret by his wife, Nadezhda Krupskaya, after a stroke had left him paralyzed and unable to speak just a month before the Party Congress. After his death in January 1924, Krupskaya turned the document over to Party officials, who opted to suppress it. Lenin's testament, translated in English, was published by the *New York Times* in 1926; the original would not be published in the Soviet Union until after Nikita Khrushchev had denounced Stalin at the XXth Party Congress in 1956.

The *troika* began to disintegrate in early 1925. In December that year, Kamenev publicly called for Stalin's removal from the position of General Secretary but was outvoted. In 1927, Kamenev became the official leader of the opposition. However, he had missed his chance and was arrested in 1934 — at the very start of the Great Purges — on the pretext of "moral complicity" in the assassination of the Old Bolshevik Sergey Kirov. Kamenev was tried and sentenced to five years imprisonment; soon thereafter, his sentence was extended to ten years. Finally, in 1936, he was put on trial again with 15 others on charges of forming a terrorist organization to assassinate Stalin and other Soviet leaders. The defendants were forced to confess to an assortment of crimes, including espionage, poisoning, and sabotage, just to name a few, before being pronounced guilty and executed by rifle squad in August 1936. In 1988, during *perestroika*, Kamenev and his co-defendants were formally cleared of all charges by the Soviet government.

Kameneva, Olga Davidovna (born Bronstein, a younger sister of Leon Trotsky) was the first wife of Lev Kamenev and the mother of two of his sons. Olga Davidovna was imprisoned after Kamenev's trial and, in September 1941, was executed together with 160 other prominent political prisoners in Medvedev forest outside the city of Oryol, 220 miles south-west of Moscow. Both her sons — Yura, 17, mentioned in the story above, and Alexander, 33, an Air Force officer — were also executed.

Molotov, Vyacheslav Mikhailovich was a Soviet politician and diplomat and a leading figure in the Soviet government up until 1957 when he was dismissed by Nikita Khrushchev. He was the principal Soviet signatory of the Nazi-Soviet non-aggression pact of 1939 (also known as the Molotov-Ribbentrop Pact). Molotov's relationship with Stalin deteriorated when Stalin arrested Molotov's wife, Polina Zhemchuzhina. Stalin advised Molotov to divorce her and even offered to find him a new wife, which Molotov firmly declined. Zhemchuzhina was released after Stalin's death. Despite tensions between him and Stalin, Molotov strongly opposed Khrushchev's policy of destalinization and defended Stalin's legacy until his own death in 1986.

Uborevich, Jeronim Petrovich was a top-ranking Soviet military commander. Arrested during the Great Purges of the Red Army, he was tried by the NKVD in May 1937, sentenced to death and executed in June 1937 at the age of 40. Like many others, he was posthumously rehabilitated in 1957.

Voroshilov, Kliment Yefremovich, who hosted the dinner party on November 8, 1932, was a Soviet military officer and politician. He was one of the first five Marshals of the Soviet Union (the highest military rank in the Soviet Union) and a full member of Stalin's Politburo. He lived in the Kremlin at the barracks of the Horse Guards. Voroshilov played a central role in Stalin's Great Purges of the late 1930s, denouncing his own military colleagues and personally signing hundreds of execution lists.

Zhemchuzhina, Polina Semyonovna was the wife of Vyacheslav Molotov, a close friend of Stalin's wife, Nadezhda Alliluyeva, and likely the last person (except possibly Stalin himself) to see Alliluyeva alive, which earned her Stalin's undying hatred. Seeking a pretext to arrest Zhemchuzhina in the late 1930s, Stalin ordered the NKVD to torture the victims of his Great Purges to extract confessions implicating Zhemchuzhina in espionage. He suspended his vendetta in 1939 after Molotov had been appointed Minister of Foreign Affairs and had signed the Molotov-Ribbentrop Pact. The Politburo sided with Molotov, declaring the allegations of sabotage and espionage against Zhemchuzhina slanderous. However, Zhemchuzhina's Jewish and foreign associations finally gave Stalin his opening in 1948. Fluent in Yiddish, Zhemchuzhina acted as translator to Golda Meir during the latter's visit to Moscow as the first Israeli envoy to the Soviet Union. She became friendly with Meir. Zhemchuzhina also actively supported the Jewish Anti-Fascist Committee (JAC) and was friendly with many of its leading members, including the great actor Solomon Mikhoels, who was murdered in 1948 on Stalin's orders. Zhemchuzhina's brother, Sam Carp, was a successful businessman in the USA. These facts supplied the necessary pretext for Stalin to have her arrested for treason in December 1948 and then convicted and sentenced to five years in a labor camp. Before Stalin's death in 1953, she was brought to Moscow in connection with the Doctors' Plot, where Stalin had planned to conduct a staged trial of Jewish doctors. It is quite possible that she was to be executed together with the doctors. The trial never took place because Stalin died days before its scheduled date. After Stalin's death in March 1953, Polina Zhemchuzhina was released and reunited with Molotov. She died of natural causes in 1970.

Index

Printed in the United States
By Bookmasters